D1172714

Boxing and Medicine

Robert C. Cantu, MD
Emerson Hospital and
National Center for Catastrophic Sports Injury Research

Editor

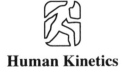

Human Kinetics

Library of Congress Cataloging-in-Publication Data

Boxing and medicine / Robert C. Cantu, editor.
  p.   cm.
  Includes index.
  ISBN 0-87322-797-2
  1. Boxing injuries.   2. Boxing injuries--Prevention.   I. Cantu,
  Robert C.
  RC1220.B6B69   1995
  617.1'027--dc20   94-33961
                                                                 CIP

ISBN: 0-87322-797-2

Copyright © 1995 by Robert C. Cantu

All rights reserved. Except for use in a review, the reproduction or utilization of this work in any form or by any electronic, mechanical, or other means, now known or hereafter invented, including xerography, photocopying, and recording, and in any information storage and retrieval system, is forbidden without the written permission of the publisher.

Developmental Editor: Patricia Sammann; **Assistant Editors:** Anna Curry, Julie Marx Ohnemus, and Henry Woolsey; **Editorial Assistant:** Karen Grieves; **Copyeditor:** Joyce Sexton; **Proofreader:** Karen Bojda; **Indexer:** Barbara Cohen; **Typesetting and Layout:** Julie Overholt; **Text Designer:** Judy Henderson; **Cover Designer:** Jack Davis; **Printer:** Braun-Brumfield

Printed in the United States of America
10 9 8 7 6 5 4 3 2 1

Human Kinetics
P.O. Box 5076, Champaign, IL 61825-5076
1-800-747-4457

Canada: Human Kinetics, Box 24040,
Windsor, ON N8Y 4Y9
1-800-465-7301 (in Canada only)

Europe: Human Kinetics, P.O. Box IW14,
Leeds LS16 6TR, England
(44) 532 781708

Australia: Human Kinetics, 2 Ingrid Street,
Clapham 5062, South Australia
(08) 371 3755

New Zealand: Human Kinetics, P.O. Box 105-231,
Auckland 1
(09) 309 2259

This book is dedicated to two former outstanding amateur boxers whose adult lives after college graduation have been largely devoted to improving boxing safety.

In the ring, the referee is the guardian of the boxer. No referee has contributed more to the profession than Arthur L. Mercante. While his accomplishments in boxing are too numerous to mention, this World Boxing Hall of Fame member is most known as the referee of more world championship matches (95) than any other.

No one has contributed more to boxing than Steve Acunto. Though remembered as a welterweight who fought in exhibitions with Barney Ross and Henry Armstrong, among others, he is better known as college boxing coach at Sarah Lawrence, Concordia College, Westchester Community College, and, for over 20 years, at the White Plains YMCA. His lasting monument, however, was the formation, with Rocky Marciano in 1969, of a nonprofit organization, The American Association for the Improvement of Boxing, devoted to improving the safety of boxing, elevating the image of the sport, and aiding the welfare of all boxers.

Contents

Contributors

Editor
Robert C. Cantu, MA, MD
Chief, Neurosurgery Service
Director, Service of Sports Medicine
Emerson Hospital, Concord, MA
and
Medical Director
National Center for Catastrophic Sports Injury Research

Joseph J. Estwanik, MD
Chairman, Sportsmedicine Committee, USA Boxing
and
Orthopedic Surgeon
Sports Science Centre
Charlotte, NC

Walter F. Stewart, PhD, MPH
Department of Epidemiology
School of Hygiene and Public Health
The Johns Hopkins University
Baltimore, MD

Barry Gordon, MD, PhD
Department of Cognitive Sciences
The Johns Hopkins University
Baltimore, MD

Vincent J. Giovinazzo, MD
Assistant Clinical Professor of Ophthalmology
State University of New York
Health Science Center
Brooklyn, NY
and
Director of Ophthalmology
Staten Island University Hospital
and
Member of Medical Advisory Board
New York State Athletic Commission

David J. Smith, MD
Attending Surgeon, Cataract and Primary Eye Care Service
Wills Eye Hospital
Philadelphia, PA

Paul F. Vinger, MD
Director, New England Eye Center
Associate Clinical Professor of Ophthalmology
Tufts University School of Medicine
Concord, MA

Francis G. O'Connor, MD
Director, Primary Care Sports Medicine
Dewitt Army Community Hospital
Clinical Assistant Professor, Family Medicine
Uniformed Services University of the Health Sciences
Bethesda, MD

Kevin W. Wildes, SJ, PhD
Assistant Professor
Philosophy Department
Georgetown University
Washington, DC
and
Senior Research Scholar
Kennedy Institute of Ethics and the Center for Clinical Bioethics
Georgetown University
Washington, DC

Loïc J.D. Wacquant, PhD
Department of Sociology
The University of California–Berkeley
and
Center for European Sociology
College de France
Paris

Barry D. Jordan, MD
Medical Director
New York State Athletic Commission
New York, NY
and
Assistant Professor of Neurology and Public Health
Cornell University Medical College
New York, NY
and
Assistant Attending Neurologist
The New York Hospital
New York, NY

Preface

Boxing is a controversial sport that has drawn criticism from physicians since its inception around 800 B.C. There is no doubt that boxing is a dangerous activity that can result in death or brain damage—but is it any more dangerous than other risky sports? For example, the chance of fatality in boxing is 1.3 per 100,000 participants. This is a fraction of the risk seen in other socially accepted sporting pursuits such as college football (3 per 100,000), motorcycle racing (7), scuba diving (11), mountaineering (51), hang gliding (55), sky diving (123), and horse racing (128) (1). In fact, studies by Gonzales (2) and Refshauge (3) suggest that the fatality rate is low in boxing compared to other sports and is continuing to decrease (4).

Brain damage also is a risk of boxing. Martland (5) introduced the term "punch-drunk" into the medical literature in 1928 when he described its occurrence in boxers; however, it may occur in anyone subjected to repeated blows to the head, and it has been reported in those who participate in soccer, football, rugby, and horse racing.

Since Martland's article appeared, many retrospective studies of boxers have been done using either pathological postmortem studies, EEGs, head CT or MRI scans, or neuropsychological tests to demonstrate chronic brain damage in former boxers. These studies show unequivocally that repeated brain injury of concussive or even subconcussive force results in characteristic patterns of brain damage and a steady decline in the ability to process information efficiently (6-11). Furthermore, the effects of repeated head injury are cumulative; this can be shown immediately at the time of the second injury. A recent study showed an alarmingly high degree of morbidity 3 months after what appeared to be seemingly insignificant head injuries (12). Although some blows to the head may be more severe than others, none are trivial, and each has the potential to be lethal.

From this medical evidence, and perhaps personal bias, a sentiment for abolishing boxing has evolved in the medical community. This sentiment peaked in January 1983 when two fiery editorials appeared in the *Journal of the American Medical Association* calling boxing an obscenity and crying for its abolition. In that same issue was a report from an AMA panel formed in 1982, which included professors of neurology and neurosurgery, that had reviewed all the medical evidence on boxing. Rather than call for a ban on boxing, the group made eight recommendations to improve boxing safety. Despite this panel's report, however, the House of Delegates at the June 1983 AMA annual meeting adopted a resolution calling for the "elimination of boxing from amateur, scholastic, intercollegiate, and governmental athletic programs" (13). More recently, the American Academy of Pediatrics and the American Academy of Neurology have voiced similar sentiments (14, 15).

Should physicians then support or reject boxing? The controversy continues, providing the rationale for the creation of this book, *Boxing and Medicine*. It is meant to provide physicians in sports medicine and related specialties with valid information on the physical dangers of boxing, the ethical and social arguments for and against boxing, and the steps that can be taken to improve boxing's safety. Readers then can decide for themselves whether to aid in making boxing safer, either by serving as a ringside physician or by supporting reforms in boxing, or to call for its abandonment.

Part I includes chapters 1 and 2 and supplies background information on the history of the relationship between boxing and medicine and the major differences between amateur and professional boxing. Part II, which includes chapters 3 through 7, provides a review of information on boxing injuries. Part III, which includes chapters 8 and 9, addresses the physician's relationship to the sport and the ethical and social ramifications of boxing. Finally, Part IV, which comprises chapters 10 and 11, offers concrete, practical recommendations about boxing and addresses the AMA's position statement to ban the sport. It includes guidelines for participants in the sport and recommendations to sports physicians serving boxers. A conclusion from the editor sums it all up at the end.

We hope that this book supplies you with the data and information you need to take a stand on boxing. If you are not supportive of boxing, then you will at least have considered the evidence fairly; and if you are supportive, we hope you will join us in continuing to try to improve safety and reduce injuries for those engaged in the ancient art of boxing.

References

1. Some high risk sports. Sporting News. 1980 Aug. 16.
2. Gonzales, T.A. Fatal injuries in competitive sports. JAMA 146:1506-1511; 1951.
3. Refshauge, J.G.H. The medical aspects of boxing. Med. J. Aust. 1:611-613; 1963.
4. Ryan, A.J. Intracranial injuries resulting from boxing. In: Mosby, T., ed. Athletic Injuries to the Head, Face, and Neck. Chicago: Year Book Inc.; 1991:p. 31-40.
5. Martland, H.S. Punch drunk. JAMA 91:1103-1107; 1928.

6. Gronwall, D.; Wrightson, P. Delayed recovery of intellectual function after minor head injury. Lancet 2:605-609; 1974.

7. Gronwall, D. Paced auditory serial-addition task: a measure of recovery from concussion. Percept. Mot. Skills 44:367-373; 1977.

8. Gronwall, D.; Wrightson, P. Duration of posttraumatic amnesia after mild head injury. J. Clin. Neuropsychol. 2:51-56; 1980.

9. Gronwall, D.; Wrightson, P. Memory and information processing capacity after closed head injury. J. Neurol. Neurosurg. Psychiatry 44:889-895; 1981.

10. Gronwall, D.; Wrightson, P. Cumulative effect of concussion. Lancet 2:995-997; 1975.

11. Symonds, C. Concussion and its sequelae. Lancet 1:1-5; 1962.

12. Rimel, R.W.; Bruno-Giordani, N.P.; Barth, J.T.; Boll, T.J.; Jane, J.A. Disability caused by minor head injury. Neurosurg. 9:221-228; 1981.

13. Lundberg, G.D. Boxing should be banned in civilized countries. JAMA 251:2696-2697; 1984.

14. Committee on Sports Medicine. Participation in boxing among children and young adults. Pediatrics 74:311-312; 1984.

15. Richards, N.G. Boxing: the intent is wrong. Va. Med. 112:122-123; 1985.

PART I

AN OVERVIEW OF BOXING

This introductory part gives the reader background information as a context for the rest of the book.

In chapter 1, Dr. Cantu highlights 20th-century events important to the relationship between boxing and medicine. Medical findings about the results of brain injury incurred during boxing have led some physicians, as well as the U.S. government, to try to control or eliminate boxing. The most heated opposition occurred during the early 1980s, when some key AMA members came out in favor of a ban on both amateur and professional boxing.

In chapter 2, Dr. Estwanik briefly outlines the major differences between amateur and professional boxing. The two types of boxing are unlike each other in many ways, from their underlying philosophy to the details of scoring, appropriate gear, and safety procedures. As safety has been given much more attention in amateur boxing than in the professional game, the potential to improve professional boxing by adopting some of the rules of amateur boxing is great.

CHAPTER **1**

Medicine's Stand on Boxing in the 20th Century

Robert C. Cantu

Medicine has affected boxing in various ways during this century through scientific, legal, and societal means. Most of the effects have been negative as individuals have sought either to restrain the practice of boxing or to develop evidence of boxing's damaging effects on the brain. But is this the role medicine should be playing, or can medicine be more helpful by encouraging safer procedures and supervising the sport? One way to assess this is to look at what has happened so far.

The Robert Fitzsimmons Case

Perhaps the earliest example of physicians influencing events in boxing occurred in 1913. Robert Fitzsimmons, who became the light-heavyweight champion of the world in 1902 at the age of 40 and held the title until 1905, lost his court battle to continue to earn a living in the only way he knew. The New York State Athletic Commission, acting upon medical advice and other factors, removed the boxing license of the former champion. Fitzsimmons sued, but the court ruled that allowing him to continue meant risking serious injury not only to himself but also to boxing and society (1).

Martland's Definition of "Punch-Drunk"

Most would say that the pioneering studies of Dr. Harrison Martland on the physical effects of boxing in the 1920s, culminating with his classic

3

paper in the *Journal of the American Medical Association* (*JAMA*) in 1928 (2; p. 1103), started the medical debate on boxing (3). In that 1928 article, he coined the term *punch-drunk* and described it as follows:

> For some time fight fans and promoters have recognized a peculiar condition occurring among prize fighters which, in ring parlance, they speak of as "punch drunk." Fighters in whom the early symptoms are well recognized are said by the fans to be "cuckoo," "goofy," "cutting paper dolls," or "slug nutty."
>
> The early symptoms of punch drunk usually appear in the extremities. There may be only an occasional and very slight flopping of one foot or leg in walking, noticeable only at intervals; or a slight unsteadiness of gait or uncertainty in equilibrium. These may not seriously interfere with fighting. In fact, many who have only these early symptoms fight extremely well, and the slight staggering may be noticed only as they walk to their corners.
>
> In some cases periods of slight mental confusion may occur as well as distinct slowing of muscular action. The early symptoms of punch drunk are well known to fight fans, and the gallery gods often shout "Cuckoo" at a fighter. I know of one fight that was stopped by the referee because he thought one of the fighters intoxicated.
>
> Many cases remain mild in nature and do not progress beyond this point. In others a very distinct dragging of the leg may develop, and with this there is a general slowing down in muscular movements, a peculiar mental attitude characterized by hesitancy in speech, tremors of the hands, and nodding movements of the head, necessitating withdrawal from the ring.
>
> Later on, in severe cases, there may develop a peculiar tilting of the head, a marked dragging of one or both legs, a staggering, propulsive gait with the facial characteristics of the Parkinsonian syndrome, or a backward swaying of the body, tremors, vertigo and deafness. Finally, marked mental deterioration may set in, necessitating commitment to an asylum.*

Martland believed that symptoms appeared in up to half of all veteran boxers. Martland, using information taken from a newspaper article, personalized and enlivened his article with this final paragraph about Gene Tunney.

---

*From "Punch Drunk" by H.S. Martland, 1928, *Journal of the American Medical Association*, **91**, pp. 1103-1107. Copyright 1928 by the American Medical Association. Reprinted by permission.

In discussing his retirement from the prize ring, Gene Tunney said in connection with his training for the second Dempsey fight: "I went into a clinch with my head down, something I never do. I plunged forward, and my partner's head came up and butted me over the left eye, cutting and dazing me badly. Then . . . he stepped back and swung his right against my jaw with every bit of his power. It landed flush and stiffened me where I stood. . . . That is the last thing I remembered for two days. They tell me that I finished out the round, knocking the man out." Tunney further stated that it was forty-eight hours before he knew who he was, and not until the seventh round of the Dempsey fight was he entirely normal. In concluding, he said: "From that incident was born my desire to quit the ring forever, the first opportunity that presented itself. . . . But most of all, I wanted to leave the game that had threatened my sanity before I met with an accident in a real fight with six ounce gloves that would permanently hurt my brain."*

Roberts's and Corsellis's Studies of Brain Injury

Over the next half century, multiple retrospective studies of predominantly professional boxers appeared that supported Martland's views.

A.H. Roberts, who reported on 224 professional boxers registered with the British Board of Boxing Control between 1929 and 1955, found a similar "dose response." Overall, 17% of cases showed chronic neurological damage attributable to boxing, and the "prevalence of injury increased with increasing boxing exposure" (4).

Dr. J.A. Nicholas Corsellis headed a team of British researchers at Runwell Hospital in Essex, England, who analyzed the brains of 15 deceased boxers and supplemented this research with interviews with the families and associates of boxers. They documented four types of brain damage that they correlated with behavioral changes (5, 6).

The most common and easily observed condition was a marked tearing and separation of the septum pellucidum between the third ventricle. The average cava of the boxers was 5.17 mm, compared with an average of 1.6 mm in 142 nonboxers. Corsellis correlated this structural change with emotional lability and especially rage reactions, which were confirmed by history in almost all the boxers.

The second structural change noted in 10 of 15 boxers was a scarring of the undersurface of the cerebellum. The force of the blows had caused

---

*From "Punch Drunk" by H.S. Martland, 1928, *Journal of the American Medical Association*, **91**, pp. 1103-1107. Copyright 1928 by the American Medical Association. Reprinted by permission.

the cerebellum to be forced down through the foramen magnum, leading to cerebellar scarring. The cerebellar injury was associated with slurred speech, a broad-based gait, and a slowing of motor movement.

Corsellis also found that this degenerative condition in some cases continued to progress long after the boxing career had ended. Most brains examined showed a third change, a decrease in pigment of the substantia nigra, a condition seen in Parkinson's syndrome. Four boxers who had difficulty with tremor and rigidity of the limbs actually were hospitalized with a diagnosis of Parkinson's syndrome.

The fourth pathological change was the prevalence of neurofibrillary tangles, especially in the medial temporal lobe. This condition is usually seen in the elderly in association with senile plaques. The tangles were seen in 14 of 15 boxers' brains, 9 of which had no senile plaques. This led Corsellis to conclude they had been caused by repeated blows to the head rather than senility.

Corsellis's boxers' brains included those of two world champions and four regional or national champions. The most successful boxers had the most brain damage. Corsellis reasoned that this was because they had the longest careers, fought the toughest opponents, and thus took the most blows to the head.

Governmental Intervention

These studies and others (which will be discussed in greater detail in chapter 3) led to extremely strict supervision of amateur boxing and a permanent ban on professional boxing in Sweden from 1969 on and in Norway from 1982 on, as well as a temporary ban in Connecticut from 1965 to 1969 (7).

Shocked by the deaths of two professional boxers in consecutive months (Willie Classen on November 23, 1979, and Tony Thomas on December 22, 1979) and one later the next year (Cleveland Denny on June 20, 1980), Congress held hearings on federal regulation of professional boxing in 1980. Edward P. Beard, then Chairman of the House Subcommittee on Labor Standards, proposed a bill to establish a federal boxing board that would register and rate all boxers, regulate medical and safety standards, and give the ring physician authority to stop a fight (8). Unfortunately, though well intended with meaningful recommendations, these congressional hearings, like all those before and since, led to stalemate and inaction.

The Medical Community's Call
for a Ban on Boxing

It has been the American Medical Association (AMA), perhaps by virtue of its size and prestige, that has to date produced the greatest stir over boxing.

An AMA advisory panel composed of preeminent physicians, including neurologists and neurosurgeons, concluded in 1983 (9), as a similar group had concluded in 1962 (10), that banning boxing was impractical and unwarranted. Instead, the panel recommended a number of safety reforms (to be discussed in chapter 11). In the same issue that carried the advisory panel's scientific report were two incendiary editorials (11, 12), one by the editor of *JAMA*, George Lundberg, calling for the abolition of boxing. On June 23, 1983, the House of Delegates of the AMA passed a resolution to publicize the harmful effects of boxing, encourage the elimination of amateur boxing, and develop legislation to curtail all boxing (13).

In May 1984 George Lundberg wrote and ran his second editorial calling for a ban on boxing (13). This was followed in December 1984 by the passage of a resolution by the House of Delegates at the AMA interim meeting calling for the elimination of amateur and professional boxing.

In 1986 George Lundberg wrote a third editorial calling for a ban on boxing, further igniting the controversy. In that editorial he noted that, as the U.S. delegates at the December 1984 meeting represented all 50 states and 54 specialty organizations, and as the medical associations of Britain, Canada, and Australia also had adopted antiboxing resolutions, "we have seen the development of a broad international medical consensus that boxing should be abolished" (14; p. 2483). This, of course, was his interpretation, and this issue has never been put to the vote of the AMA membership.

To support its ban on boxing, the AMA's House of Delegates called for the AMA to launch a three-part attack:

1. To communicate the AMA's opposition to boxing to regulating bodies such as the USA/Amateur Boxing Federation
2. To provide guidance to state medical societies that wished to lobby for antiboxing legislation
3. To launch a nationwide publicity campaign about the dangers of boxing

In addition to the AMA, the British, Canadian, Australian, and World Medical associations have called for a ban on boxing (15). In the August 1984 issue of *Pediatrics* (16), the American Academy of Pediatrics went on record as opposing boxing in any sports program for children. In 1985 the American Academy of Neurology went on record as opposing boxing (17, 18).

The AMA's and other organizations' ban on boxing has several faults. First, the AMA's statement was not put to the vote of the entire membership, and thus may not reflect the views of the entire membership. Second, and more important, a ban probably is not feasible in the United States now or in the future. By taking such a confrontational and adversarial position, the medical community positions itself adversely and thus loses the opportunity to facilitate changes that would make boxing safer.

References

1. Fitzsimmons v. New York State Athletic Commission, 146 NYS 117 (1914).
2. Martland, H.S. Punch drunk. JAMA 91:1103-1107; 1928.
3. Gorman, T. Death in the ring. Hygenia 385:420-421; 1949.
4. Roberts, A.H. Brain damage in boxers. London: Pitman Medical and Scientific; 1969:61-99.
5. Corsellis, J.; Bruton, C.J.; Freeman-Browne, D. The aftermath of boxing. Psychol. Med. 3:270-303; 1973.
6. Petal, M. Boxing is murder. Phy. Sportsmed. 2:67-68; 1974.
7. Ryan, A.J. Death in the ring. Phy. Sportsmed. 8:47-48; 1980.
8. Moore, M. The challenge of boxing: bringing safety to the ring. Phy. Sportsmed. 8:101-105; 1980.
9. Council on Scientific Affairs. Brain injury in boxing. JAMA 249:254-257; 1983.
10. Committee on Medical Aspects of Sports. Statement on boxing. JAMA 181:242; 1962.
11. Lundberg, G.D. Boxing should be banned in civilized countries. JAMA 249:250; 1983.
12. Van Allen, M.W. The deadly degrading sport. JAMA 249:250-251; 1983.
13. Lundberg, G.D. Boxing should be banned in civilized countries—round 2. JAMA 251:2696-2698; 1984.
14. Lundberg, G.D. Boxing should be banned in civilized countries—round 3. JAMA 255:2483-2485; 1986.
15. Morrison, R.G. Medical and public health aspects of boxing. JAMA 255:2475-2480; 1986.
16. Committee on Sports Medicine. Participation in boxing among children and young adults. Pediatrics 74:311-312; 1984.
17. Richards, N.G. Boxing: the intent is wrong. Va. Med. 112:122-123; 1985.
18. Richards, N.G. Ban boxing. Neurology 34:1485-1486; 1985.

CHAPTER 2

Professional and Amateur Rules and Regulations

Joseph J. Estwanik

How often does the informed public confuse the slick, highly skillful, on-the-mat moves of the "disciplined" amateur scholastic wrestler with the staged, high-flying, circus-like script of the long-haired professional wrestler? Not often. Why, then, the great confusion between the sport of amateur boxing and the business of professional boxing? Even such esteemed and educated groups as the American Medical Association demonstrate little knowledge of these differences, even as they are proposing legislation specifically for boxing. Hopefully the following information will help the reader separate fact from fiction, sport from business, and amateur from pro.

It can certainly be debated whether a relationship between amateur and pro is good, advisable, inevitable, or bad. A reality check does, however, reconfirm that the pathway to the "big bucks" is narrow and lonely. The economic realities of the professional business of boxing can be elucidated by the observation that in 1992 nine professional boxers earned 85% of the total monies generated by boxing in the states of New Jersey and California ($85 million). Many hundreds of itinerant pro boxers toil for peanuts while managers, promoters, trainers, and sparring partners stand in line for their share of the loot.

The general public quite often has a rather skewed and vividly sordid picture when the subject of boxing surfaces. However, the knowledgeable aficionado of amateur boxing understands his sport in a manner similar to one appreciating the reflexive moves of the amateur wrestler. Times have changed. Patriotic, glamorous events like *USA vs. Soviet Union* used to sell tickets, but present events in world politics have suppressed the ancient enemies of the United States and the thunder of nationalistic flag-waving match-ups. The blood and gore have been politely removed from the amateur ring by safety-conscious officials and well-meaning fatherlike coaches. Don't bet on which round the knockout will occur in while watching the amateurs. Headgear, limited numbers of rounds, and ever-alert referees eliminate and intercept one-sided, dangerous mismatches.

How then might we categorize the differences between amateur and professional boxing? Table 2.1 shows 12 major categories in which amateur and professional boxing differ. These 12 categories may not always show startling contrasts, but rather subtle differences. Such distinctions provide, in a very practical sense, categorizations for safety and organizational goals. It is the wish of the author that the safety innovations of amateur boxing might be applied to the professional ranks, as ongoing educational efforts deliver the scientific information for improvements in the amateur sport. The professionals should continue to incorporate the innovations developed for the dedicated amateur boxer.

Historically, those sponsoring sports have spurned classic scientific methods of analysis for injury trends based on the public health principles of epidemiology. But there are exceptions. American football was challenged by an alarming annual rise in cervical spine traumas resulting in death and catastrophic spinal cord injury to participants. Was this tradition-rich and revenue-producing favorite of youth leagues, high schools, and colleges banished from its prominence in yearbooks and weekend homecomings? Were its athletes abandoned or football programs ordered to cease and desist? Of course not.

The scientific methodologies of familiarization with the sport, statistical analysis, identification of the mechanisms of injury, and recommendations for rule and equipment changes were implemented. As a response, one critical technique was banned: "spearing" with the helmet.

Boxing was long ago dropped from the academic curriculum, which has led to a subsequent failure to implement certain modern advances of sports medicine. This penalized the sport. The athletes failed to gain the advice of university-trained coaches and trainers. Trainers, or "cut-men," were the "docs" of the ring. Tradition was a heavyweight and science a welterweight.

As the bell rings, organized medicine and its sports medicine experts are challenged. Maybe we're behind in points, but let's make this a big round. Act as a coach—analyze the opponents, come up with the right defense, and plan effective counters. But above all, don't quit on your athlete.

Table 2.1   Differences Between Amateur and Professional Boxing*

Category	Amateur	Professional
Philosophy	Amateur boxing is pure sport. The athletes compete for the thrill of athletic endeavor and to show that their prowess is greater than that of their opponents. They also sometimes compete for the U.S. against foreign competitors. Their training and experience may result in the opportunity to start a successful pro career.	Professional boxing is a business and a profession. Concern for dollars often overrides safety concerns.
Organization	All amateur boxing comes under the jurisdiction of a single, unified national governing body (NGB). As an NGB, USA Boxing has jurisdiction over the administration, eligibility, sanctioning, representation, and rules of competition for men's and women's amateur boxing in the U.S.	Many state-controlled commissions have different sets of rules. Therefore, no single, unified body exists, nor is there one single set of standard rules and guidelines.
	All amateurs nationwide are registered with USA Boxing.	No single nationwide registry exists. Registry is controlled locally.
International rules	Amateur boxing uses the same set of rules worldwide. The U.S. conforms to these rules plus more stringent rules in some areas for safety.	Professional boxing has three sets of rules—WBA, WBC, and those set by state commissions.
Rulebooks	A single rulebook contains specific rules that govern or regulate a point or area.	Many rulebooks exist, but none is complete or is used universally.

(continued)

*From "Categorized Differences Between Amateur and Professional Boxing," n.d., Colorado Springs: USA Boxing. Copyright by USA Boxing. Adapted by permission.

Table 2.1 *(continued)*

Category	Amateur	Professional
Scoring	a. In amateur boxing, the force of a blow or its effect on the opponent does not count. Therefore, the knockout is a by-product in amateur boxing. The main objective is to score points. A blow that knocks a boxer to the mat receives no more points than a regular blow. A knockdown is scored as a single blow and does not necessarily make the boxer the winner of that round.	a. Added "weight" is given to a blow based on its impact and effect on the opponent. Therefore, the knockout is an objective in the pros. In rare cases, a boxer who scores a knockdown may lose the round.
	b. A blow counts for scoring only if the knuckle surface is used. Slapping or other types of blows are not allowed or counted for points. Therefore, the striking area is limited to the knuckle of the fist and must hit the front and side of the head and body and above the waist.	b. Not as much attention is given to the placement of scoring blows.
Rounds	Bouts are three 3-minute rounds, with a 1-minute break between each round. For Junior Olympic boxers, rounds are graduated in length from 1 minute to 2 minutes, depending on the age group.	Championship bouts have either 12 or 15 rounds. Other bouts vary from 4 to 10 rounds. Rounds last 3 minutes.

Category	Amateur	Professional
Safety during the competition	a. A mouthpiece is required. It must be worn at all times; if it falls out, it is immediately replaced.	a. A mouthpiece is worn.
	b. Headgear is required.	b. Headgear is prohibited.
	c. Boxers receive standing 8-counts. This is a safety precaution, as it gives the referee 8 seconds to evaluate the condition of the boxer. Based on the referee's decision, the bout may continue or be stopped.	c. Certain pro world bodies have recently adopted the standing 8-count.
	d. In case of injury, the referee stops the bout and takes the boxer to the corner for the doctor to examine and evaluate. Based on the doctor's evaluation, the bout may continue or be stopped.	d. Under some rules, it is the same.
	e. More control is exercised by the referee in the ring. The referee gives cautions to a boxer to let him know that he is violating fundamentals and rules.	e. The referee warns boxers only for a "harm-foul, blow-type" infraction, not for technique.
	f. The referee will stop the bout if a boxer is outclassed.	f. The referee is authorized to stop a bout if a boxer is outclassed, but rarely does so due to financial and TV arrangements.

(continued)

Table 2.1 *(continued)*

Category	Amateur	Professional
Safety during the competition *(continued)*	g. The criteria for stopping bouts due to injury are stricter. For example, lacerations or swelling that blocks vision will cause the bout to be stopped.	g. Rules are less strict with respect to which injuries will stop a bout. For example, a boxer can continue to box if his eye is swollen shut or if a cut around the eye, nose, or mouth is bleeding badly.
	h. The use of the head (butting) is strictly regulated. The boxer is cautioned but then may be warned or lose points if he continues to butt.	h. Butting is laxly controlled.
	i. The bell cannot "save" a boxer from a knockout or stopped contest. The count continues to completion, regardless of when the bell rings, except in the finals of a tournament, such as the Olympics, Pan Am Games, or U.S. Championships.	i. A boxer can be "saved" from a knockout or stopped contest by the ringing of the bell in some states.
Gloves	a. In the U.S., all boxers use 10- or 12-ounce gloves. Boxers weighing 106-156 pounds wear 10-ounce gloves; boxers weighing 165-201 pounds or more wear 12-ounce gloves.	a. All boxers use 8-ounce gloves.
	b. Gloves have been designed to absorb, not transmit, shock.	b. Gloves have been designed to transmit force except in rare instances; groups are trying to improve glove design.

Category	Amateur	Professional
Gloves (continued)	c. The striking surface is indicated by a white area to aid judges in scoring.	c. The striking surface is not marked.
Appearance	a. A boxer wears a top to aid in identification, absorb sweat and dirt, and keep gloves cleaner.	a. Boxers do not wear tops.
	b. No foreign substance is permitted on the body, as is used in "greasing up."	b. Boxers are allowed to "grease up."
	c. A boxer may not wear a beard or goatee; a thin, pencil-line moustache is allowed. Hair may not impair vision.	c. No such rules exist.
Physical exams	a. A pre-bout physical is conducted before each bout. In a tournament, boxers receive an initial physical and then have one each day they compete. Post-bout evaluations are conducted as the boxers exit the ring.	a. The practice is the same.
	b. If a bout is stopped because of blows to the head, the boxer is not allowed to compete or work out in the gym for 4 weeks. He must then be certified by a physician to return. For suspensions greater than 4 weeks, the boxer must be cleared by additional tests.	b. The practice is often the same, but not in all cases. It depends on state regulations.
Study groups	USA Boxing study groups are constantly trying to improve equipment, rules, and techniques. The safety of the boxer is always foremost.	Some groups attempt to improve professional boxing, but there is no unified, concentrated effort.

(continued)

Table 2.1 *(continued)*

Category	Amateur	Professional
Seminars and clinics	Seminars and clinics are held to train and educate officials and coaches. Symposiums are also held for officials, physicians, coaches, etc., to study and discuss the most up-to-date techniques and styles.	Some groups attempt to train and educate, but there is no unified, concentrated effort.

PART II

THE MEDICAL RISKS OF BOXING

What are the true medical risks of boxing? Many studies exist in the literature, but almost all have been retrospective and cross-sectional in design. Almost none of them have been carried out by sports medicine professionals who are knowledgeable of the relative injury risks in all sports. And few studies, especially those for head injury, control for the possibilities of head injury outside the ring, substance abuse, and aging.

This part, written by medical professionals, takes a look at the possible medical risks associated with boxing and at the existing literature. Each chapter on injuries was created by someone with expertise in that area: a neurosurgeon writes about head injury; an ophthalmologist writes about eye injuries. How this information is put into practice is explained in the final chapter on the ringside physician's role.

In chapter 3 Dr. Cantu covers brain injuries, an area of great interest in boxing. He discusses the common mechanisms of brain injury in boxing and describes possible types of acute and chronic injuries. This topic is further probed in chapter 4, which presents a study by Drs. Stewart and Gordon exploring the question of whether amateur boxing, as opposed to professional boxing, holds a significant risk of brain injury for participants. It seems to show that some changes to the brain do occur, but not to a clinically significant extent.

Chapter 5 moves to the area of eye injuries, another frequent result of boxing. In this chapter Drs. Giovinazzo, Smith, and Vinger describe possible eye and visual injuries, attempt to ascertain the incidence of such injuries in boxers, and make some suggestions on how to prevent eye injuries in boxing.

Chapter 6 looks at other injuries likely to result from boxing. Beginning with an analysis of the incidence and relative frequency of various types of injuries, Dr. Estwanik then goes on to describe the mechanisms and symptoms of these injuries. They include injuries to the upper and lower extremities, the trunk, and the head and face.

In the final chapter, chapter 7, Drs. Estwanik and O'Connor describe the role of the physician in boxing. For those who have not served in such a position, they describe the preparticipation exam, the ringside responsibilities, and the post-bout evaluation. Their account of the ringside physician's duties shows how the physician can improve safety and reduce the effects of boxing injuries.

CHAPTER 3

Brain Injuries

Robert C. Cantu

Injury to the brain is the most frequent fatal catastrophic sports injury (1). As the brain is incapable of regeneration, an injury to this organ is singularly important.

Football has accounted for the most medical literature and media attention on brain injury, as well as the largest number of fatal head injuries of any sport (2). From 1973 to 1983 deaths from head injuries caused by playing football exceeded all other competitive sports fatalities from head injuries combined (2).

Boxing has been the other sport most associated with head injury. From 1918 to 1983, 645 fatalities were recorded worldwide, most in professional boxing (3). From 1979 to 1985 there were 28 deaths, suggesting a decreasing trend in the number of fatalities (4). Other sports that historically have shown a high inherent risk of head injury include horseback riding (5, 6), ice hockey (7, 8), martial arts (9), sky diving (10, 11), rugby (12), and vehicular racing (automobile, motorcycle) (13, 14).

Mechanisms of Brain Injury

There are three types of stresses that can be generated by an applied force and imparted to the brain: compressive, tensile (stretching), and shearing (a force applied parallel to a surface). Shearing stresses are extremely poorly tolerated by the brain, whereas uniform compressive stresses are tolerated reasonably well. Blunt head trauma causes shearing injury to nerve fibers and neurons in proportion to the degree the head is accelerated and these acceleration forces are imparted to the brain (15-17). Blows to the side of the head tend to produce greater acceleration and angular shearing forces than those directly to the face, while blows to the chin, which acts as a lever, produce maximal shear forces.

It is necessary to recognize three principles to understand how forces produce skull and brain injury.

1. A moving head impacting against an unyielding object usually produces maximum brain injury opposite the side of cranial impact (contre coup injury). Such lesions are most common at the tips and under surfaces of the frontal and temporal lobes.
2. A forceful blow to the resting movable head usually produces maximum brain injury beneath the point of cranial impact (coup injury).
3. If a skull fracture is present, the first two dicta do not pertain because the bone itself, usually transiently (linear skull fracture) or permanently (depressed skull fracture) displaced at the moment of impact, may directly injure brain tissue.

By converting focally applied external stresses to a more uniform compressive stress, the cerebral-spinal fluid (CSF) acts as a shock absorber, cushioning and protecting the brain. This is accomplished because the fluid follows the contours of the sulci and gyri and distributes the force uniformly. Without CSF, compressive forces would be received by the gyri crest but not in the depths of the sulci, thus setting up damaging shearing forces.

Shearing stresses may still be imparted to the brain despite the presence of CSF. Shearing forces will occur at those sites where rotational gliding is hindered if rotational forces are applied to the head. These areas are characterized by rough irregular surface contacts between the brain and skull, hindering smooth movement; dissipation of CSF between the brain and the skull; and dura mater-brain attachments impeding brain motion. It is in the frontal and temporal regions that the first condition, irregular surface contacts between the brain and skull, is most prominent. This explains why major brain contusions occur at these sites. Coup and contre coup injuries are explained by the second condition, dissipation of CSF. The brain lags toward the trailing surface when the head is accelerated prior to impact. This squeezes away the protective spinal fluid and allows the shearing forces to be maximal at this site. The brain lag actually thickens the layer of CSF under the point of impact; this thickening explains the lack of coup injury in moving head injury. On the other hand, there is neither brain lag nor disproportionate distribution of CSF when the head is stationary prior to impact. This accounts for the absence of contre coup injury in the presence of coup injury.

Finally, Newton's law that force = mass × acceleration must be appreciated. If the neck muscles are tensed at the moment of impact, an athlete's head can sustain far greater forces without brain injury. This is because the mass of the head is essentially its own weight in the relaxed state, but it approximates the mass of the body when the neck is rigidly tensed.

Acute Brain Injuries

Some of the acute brain injuries possible in boxing include concussion, intracranial hemorrhage, and second impact or malignant brain edema syndrome.

Concussion

Concussion is the most common head injury in all sports, including boxing. Universal agreement on the definition of concussion presently does not exist. The presence of retrograde or posttraumatic amnesia often is helpful in making the diagnosis, especially in mild cases. On the basis of the duration of unconsciousness or posttraumatic amnesia or both, I have developed a practical scheme for grading the severity of concussion (see Table 3.1).

Grade 1, the most mild concussion, occurs without loss of consciousness. The only neurologic deficit is a brief period of posttraumatic amnesia that may be fleeting or may last up to 30 minutes.

Grade 2, a moderate concussion, usually involves a brief period of unconsciousness not exceeding 5 minutes. It may also occur rarely with no loss of consciousness but with a protracted period of posttraumatic amnesia lasting over 30 minutes but less than 24 hours.

Grade 3, a severe concussion, occurs with a more protracted period of unconsciousness lasting over 5 minutes. Rarely it may occur without unconsciousness but with a sustained period of posttraumatic amnesia lasting longer than 24 hours.

Table 3.1 Severity of Concussion*

Grade	Symptoms
1 (mild)	No loss of consciousness; posttraumatic amnesia of 1-30 min
2 (moderate)	Loss of consciousness for less than 5 min; or posttraumatic amnesia of more than 30 min to 24 hr
3 (severe)	Loss of consciousness for 5 min or more; or posttraumatic amnesia of 24 hr or more

*From "Guidelines for Return to Contact Sports After Cerebral Concussion" by R.C. Cantu, 1986, *Physician and Sportsmedicine*, **14**, p. 76. Copyright 1986 by McGraw-Hill, Inc. Adapted by permission.

Today there is unequivocal evidence that repeated brain injury of concussive or even subconcussive force may result in characteristic patterns of
brain damage and a steady decline in one's ability to process information
efficiently (18-22). Furthermore, the effects of repeated brain injury may
be cumulative, and this can be shown immediately at the time of the
second injury, not necessarily only years later. While some blows to the
head may be more severe than others, none should be considered trivial
and each has the potential to be lethal.

Intracranial Hemorrhage

Intracranial hemorrhage is the leading cause of death from head injury
in all sports, including boxing. There are four major types of hemorrhage
to which the referee, trainer, and physician must be alert (see Table 3.2).
Since all four types of intracranial hemorrhage may be fatal, rapid and
accurate initial assessment is essential. Appropriate follow-up after an
athletic head injury is also mandatory.

The most rapidly progressive intracranial hematoma is an epidural
hematoma. This lesion occurs usually due to a fracture of the temporal
bone and results from a tear in a meningeal artery supplying the covering
(dura) of the brain. The clot accumulates inside the skull but outside the
dura of the brain. Since it arises from a torn artery, it may reach a fatal
size in 30 to 60 minutes. Characteristically, although not always, there is
a lucid interval after the initial period of unconsciousness, before the
athlete experiences increasing headache and progressive deterioration in
level of consciousness as the clot rapidly accumulates and intracranial
pressure rapidly increases. Almost always, the epidural hematoma will
become evident within an hour or two of the initial brain injury. In boxing,
this is not the most common type of intracranial hemorrhage.

The subdural hematoma, a second type of intracranial hemorrhage,
occurs between the brain surface and the dura due to a torn bridging
vein, and is the leading cause of death in boxing. Because the forces
necessary to produce a subdural hematoma due to a torn bridging vein
exceed the forces necessary to produce unconsciousness, this lesion characteristically occurs with loss of consciousness at the time the injury is
sustained. It is therefore most associated with a prolonged period of
unconsciousness following a knockout. With this injury there is also commonly associated brain tissue disruption, and this is what ultimately
determines the degree of recovery for the athlete. If a subdural hematoma
requires surgery in the first 24 hours, the mortality is significant, due not
so much to the clot itself as to the associated brain injury. A less common
form of subdural occurs over a period of days or weeks and is referred
to as a chronic subdural hematoma. In this lesion there is a torn bridging
vein but usually no brain injury per se. The individual may experience

Table 3.2 Four Types of Intracranial Hemorrhage

Type of hemorrhage	Cause	Signs/Symptoms	Pathology
Epidural hematoma	Temporal skull fracture with torn middle meningeal artery	Briefly unconscious, then lucid interval followed by headache and rapid loss of consciousness, all within 1-2 hours	Blood clot between skull and dura
Subdural hematoma	Acceleration blow to brain causing tearing of bridging cortical veins	Usually unconscious immediately with subsequent neurological deterioration from clot enlargement and/or cerebral edema	Blood clot under dura outside of brain surface
Intracerebral hematoma	Bleeding deep in the brain from a torn artery, occasionally rupture of aneurysm or arteriovenous malformation	Usually unconscious immediately with subsequent neurological deterioration from clot enlargement and/or cerebral edema	Blood clot deep in brain tissue
Subarachnoid hemorrhage	Bleeding from superficial small pial vessels. Occasionally from ruptured cerebral aneurysm or arteriovenous malformation.	Severe headache, often no loss of consciousness. Neurological deterioration may occur due to cerebral edema.	Bruise on surface of brain

a variety of cerebral symptoms, and the chronic subdural can be shown on either a CAT scan or MRI scan of the brain.

The intracerebral hematoma is the third type of intracranial hemorrhage that can be seen following head trauma in boxing. This is much less common than the first two types of hematoma discussed. It may also be due to a ruptured congenital vascular lesion such as an aneurysm or arteriovenous malformation. With intracerebral hematomas there is usually not a lucid interval, and neurologic deterioration may be extremely rapid.

A subarachnoid hemorrhage is the fourth type of brain hemorrhage that can be seen in boxing. It occurs as a result of a disruption of tiny surface blood vessels in the pia arachnoid layer on the surface of the brain. It is analogous to a bruise in muscle tissue. With this lesion there is often significant associated brain swelling. This hemorrhage can also result from a ruptured cerebral aneurysm or arteriovenous malformation.

Second Impact or Malignant Brain Edema Syndrome

Though the injury itself was first described by Richard Schneider (23), Saunders and Harbaugh in their 1984 article in the *Journal of the American Medical Association* (*JAMA*) (24) were the first to use the term *second impact* for what has since been called the Second Impact Syndrome of Catastrophic Head Injury. With this syndrome an athlete receives an initial head injury, often a concussion or possibly a more severe injury such as a cerebral contusion. After this first head injury the athlete suffers postconcussive symptoms such as a headache, difficulty in thinking, or balance, motor, or sensory symptoms. Before all of these symptoms clear, be it days or weeks later, the athlete returns to competition. After a second head blow, which may be remarkably minor, this syndrome may occur.

What pathologically happens with the second impact syndrome is a loss of autoregulation of blood supply to the brain, leading to vascular engorgement within the cranium (25, 26). This in turn produces markedly increased intracranial pressure, which leads either to herniation of the medial surface (uncus) of the temporal lobe or lobes below the tentorium or to herniation of the cerebellar tonsils through the foramen magnum. The usual time course is extremely rapid—seconds to several minutes. With brain herniation and brain stem compromise, coma ensues, often with ocular and respiratory failure.

The typical scenario in boxing is an athlete still symptomatic from a prior head injury who participates in a subsequent boxing match and receives a second head blow, often considered trivial. The athlete usually appears stunned but does not lose consciousness and often completes the given round. Then in the next period of seconds to a minute or two, the athlete rapidly deteriorates from a "dazed" state to one of deep coma. The athlete in essence deteriorates within minutes from a conscious though "stunned" state to a semicomatose state with rapidly dilating pupils, loss of eye movements, and often respiratory failure. The time from second impact to brain stem failure secondary to brain herniation (which in turn is secondary to increased intracranial pressure due to vascular engorgement of the brain) is usually only a few minutes or less. This demise is far more rapid than usually seen with an epidural hematoma.

In boxing the Second Impact Syndrome is of particular concern when a boxer is subjected to more than one match in a given day. It is also the likely cause of death in those instances in which a boxer who has sustained significant trauma throughout a match suddenly collapses at the end of the match.

Chronic Brain Injuries

Two common chronic brain injuries that occur in boxing are postconcussion syndrome and dementia pugilistica.

Postconcussion Syndrome

The postconcussion syndrome is a second late effect of concussion. This syndrome consists of headache (especially with exertion), dizziness, fatigue, irritability, and, especially, impaired memory and concentration. Its true incidence is not clearly known. The persistence of postconcussion symptoms indicates altered neurotransmitter function. This usually correlates with the duration of posttraumatic amnesia. An athlete should be evaluated with a CAT scan and neuropsychiatric testing when these symptoms persist. Return to competition must be deferred until all diagnostic studies are normal and all postconcussion symptoms have abated, or else the athlete is at risk for the highly fatal Second Impact Syndrome.

Dementia Pugilistica

The late or chronic effects of repeated head trauma of concussive or even subconcussive force lead to anatomical patterns of chronic brain injury with correlating signs and symptoms. It is perhaps such injuries, chronicled in a number of professional boxers in the world's literature, that have most concerned individuals who have called for a ban on boxing. The characteristic symptoms and signs of this traumatic encephalopathy may occur in anyone subjected to repeated blows to the head from any cause and have been described in a number of athletes in sports outside of boxing, including soccer, horse racing, automobile racing, rugby, and American football. The characteristic signs and symptoms include emotional lability with mood swings and a diminished ability to control one's temper, which may lead to violent behavior. The most prevalent mood is fatuous cheerfulness, but depression and paranoia may occur. Often memory, speech, and thought deteriorate, leading to obvious dementia. Other neurologic signs and symptoms due to basal ganglia (substantia nigra) injury include tremor, rigidity, and brachykinesis. Cerebellar injury leads to slurred speech and loss of balance and coordination (see Table 3.3).

A chronological synopsis of the salient international literature on chronic brain injury in boxers includes the following articles:

H.S. Martland introduced the term *punch-drunk* into the medical literature in 1928 (27). While described in boxers, this traumatic

Table 3.3 Four Main Components of Chronic Brain Damage (Dementia Pugilistica)

Area damaged	Clinical symptoms/signs
Septum pellicidum, adjacent periventricular grey matter, frontal and temporal lobes	Altered affect (euphoria, emotional lability) and memory
Degeneration of the substantia nigra	Parkinson's syndrome of tremor, rigidity, and brachykinesia
Cerebellar scarring and nerve cell loss	Slurred speech, loss of balance and coordination
Diffuse neuronal loss	Loss of intellect, Alzheimer's syndrome

encephalopathy may occur in anyone subjected to repeated blows to the head from any cause. Martland's now famous 1928 essay in *JAMA* (27) describes Gene Tunney's grade 3 concussion suffered in training for the second Dempsey fight, which was responsible for Tunney's retiring from the ring while still heavyweight champion. Tunney explained:

"I went into a clinch with my head down, something I never do. I plunged forward, and my partner's head came up and butted me over the left eye, cutting and dazing me badly. Then . . . he stepped back and swung his right against my jaw with every bit of his power. It landed flush and stiffened me where I stood. . . . That is the last thing I remembered for two days. They tell me that I finished out the round, knocking the man out." In concluding, he said: "From that incident was born my desire to quit the ring forever, the first opportunity that presented itself. . . . But most of all, I wanted to leave the game that had threatened my sanity before I met with an accident in a real fight with six ounce gloves that would permanently hurt my brain."*

In 1957, MacDonald Critchley reported on his experience with 69 cases of chronic neurological disease in boxers (28). His observations included the following:

1. The punch-drunk syndrome is more common among professionals than among amateurs.

---

*From "Punch Drunk" by H.S. Martland, 1928, *Journal of the American Medical Association*, **91**, pp. 1103-1107. Copyright 1928 by the American Medical Association. Reprinted by permission.

2. This syndrome is found in all weight classes, but characteristically in smaller men who might fight heavier opponents.
3. Boxers with this syndrome are known for being able to "take" a punch and absorb punishment.
4. Boxers with this syndrome are usually known as "sluggers" rather than scientific boxers and usually are second or third rate boxers.

In the same article, Critchley described what he called the "groggy state." He regarded this condition as midway between normal performance and a knockout and characterized it as "mental confusion with subsequent amnesia, together with an impairment in the speed and accuracy of the motor skill represented by the act of boxing."

Also in the same article, Critchley reviewed the published electroencephalographic experience (29, 30) of that decade and concluded that the EEG record at that time was a "less sensitive index of punch-drunkenness than . . . the clinical evidence," as he had observed symptoms and signs in subjects with normal EEG records.

Over the next decade, more case reports accumulated that documented further evidence of chronic degeneration in mental function (31-46). In 1969, at the behest of the Royal College of Physicians of London, Dr. A.H. Roberts published a monograph reviewing the medical literature to that point and presenting studies of British professional boxers (47). According to Roberts, the clinical picture of the punch-drunk syndrome in its mildest form includes some or all of several features: dysarthria, that is, problems with muscular control resembling those of Parkinson's disease; spasticity, that is, a jerky form of impaired muscle control, tremor, or shaking; and dementia, that is, a reduction in intelligence.

The following year, Friedrich Unterharnscheidt published a massive review of the historical and medical aspects of boxing in which, in addition to an exhaustive review of the medical literature published at that time, he reported original scientific measurements of forces applied to the head in boxing with gloves of varying weights. He commented that "every boxer must expect permanent traumatic damage which is greater the earlier he begins to box, the more frequently he participates, and the longer his career" (48).

It remained for Dr. J.A. Nicholas Corsellis and his colleagues to describe postmortem findings in the brains of men who had been boxers (49). They described a characteristic pattern of cerebral change that appeared to be the result not only of the boxing but also of changes in the septum pellucidum, a partition in the middle of the brain that may shear into two layers or even be shredded by the distortions of the brain that follow blows to the head (see Figure 3.1). They found destruction of the limbic system, a portion of the brain that governs emotion and has a role in memory and learning. There was a characteristic loss of cells from the cerebellum, a part of the brain that governs balance and coordination.

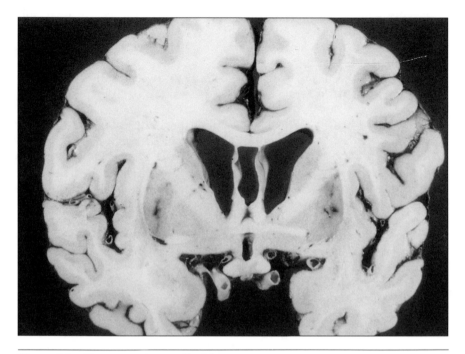

Figure 3.1 Cavum septum pellucidum.

Finally, there was an unusual microscopic change widespread throughout the brain resembling changes that occur with Alzheimer's, a disease which causes progressive loss of intelligence, but differing sufficiently (neurofibrillary tangles only and no senile plaques) to be regarded as a distinct, different entity unique to subjects suffering repeated blows to the head.

Structural changes in the brains of boxers during life were identified as early as 1962 when Spillane (46) drew particular attention to the cavum septum pellucidum, which he had outlined in air encephalograms of four of his five patients. Air encephalograms involve the injection of air into the spinal fluid compartment surrounding the brain and at the time were the only means of showing the shape of the brain on x-rays. The tests were painful, generally required hospitalization, and had some potential for harm. As a result, they were not widely used.

With the advent of the computed tomographic (CT) scanner and more recently the magnetic resonance (MR) scanner, there is now an innocuous, painless, outpatient means to identify the same changes that used to be diagnosed by means of air encephalography. Utilizing the CT scan, recent studies have documented characteristic changes in currently practicing boxers. One report concludes that the "data show that boxers with even a moderate number of bouts may suffer cerebral atrophy" (50; p. 213).

Furthermore, the authors found that the degree of cerebral atrophy corresponded with the number of bouts in which the subject had been a participant. A second article, which reported on 10 professional boxers, confirmed these findings (51). A third report, which gave less detail than the others, also indicated changes in four of six professional boxers studied (41).

Critical Analysis of Prior Studies of Chronic Brain Injury in Boxers

While all of the studies previously cited do document cerebral injury in athletes who once boxed, one must exercise caution in making causal inference from these studies about the risks in boxing. All were retrospective and cross-sectional in design. Thus, it is not certain whether in each case the structural or behavioral changes preceded or followed boxing-related experiences. They could be attributed to factors other than boxing, such as drug abuse, alcoholism, or accidents.

All these studies are further limited by the absence of an appropriate control or comparison group. Some clinicians may maintain that, when using standardized tests such as an EEG, CT scan, microscopy of the brain, or neuropsychological tests, a control group is not necessary because a comparison is being made with the general population. This reasoning is fallacious. It is based on the assumption that an individual clinician deals with a wide range of patients, when in reality most physicians have very select patient populations. It also assumes that boxers are representative of the population when in truth they are a very select group. The appropriate group for comparison is one in which similar selection factors operate, such as age- and gender-matched siblings.

Other design flaws of many of these studies relate to the sensitivity of the measures used, the subjective interpretation of data such as an EEG, and often the inadequate size of the study group.

References

1. Mueller, F.O.; Schindler, R.D. Annual survey of football injury research 1931-1986. Kansas City, MO: American Football Coaches Assoc., NCAA, and Nat. Fed. of State High School Assoc.; 1987.
2. Kraus, J.F.; Conroy, C. Mortality and morbidity from injuries in sports and recreation. Ann. Rev. Public Health 5:163-192; 1984.
3. Putnam, P. Going-going-gone. Sports Illus. 1983 June 6:23-46.
4. Ryan, A.J. Intracranial injuries resulting from boxing (1918-1989). Clin. Sports Med. 6:31-39; 1987.
5. Barclay, W.R. Equestrian sports. JAMA 240:1892-1893; 1978.
6. Barber, H.M. Horse-play: survey of accidents with horses. Br. Med. J. 3:532-534; 1973.

7. Hussey, H.H. Ice hockey injuries. JAMA 236:187; 1976.

8. Fekite, J.F. Severe brain injury and death following rigid hockey accidents. The effectiveness of the 'safety helmets' of amateur hockey players. Can. Med. Assoc. J. 99:1234-1239; 1968.

9. McLatchie, G.R.; Davies, J.E.; Caulley, J.H. Injuries in karate, a case for medical control. J. Trauma 2:956-958; 1980.

10. Krel, F.W. Parachuting for sport—study of 100 deaths. JAMA 194:264-268; 1965.

11. Petras, A.F.; Hoffman, E.P. Roentgenographic skeletal injury patterns in parachute jumping. Am. J. Sports Med. 11:325-328; 1983.

12. McCoy, G.F.; Piggot, J.; Macafee, A.L.; Adair, I.V. Injuies of the cervical spine in schoolboy rugby football. J. Bone Joint Surg. 66B(4):500-503; 1984.

13. Bodnar, L.M. Sports medicine with reference to back and neck injuries. Curr. Pract. Orthop. Surg. 7:116-153; 1977.

14. Clarke, K.; Braslow, A. Football fatalities in actuarial perspective. Med. Sci. Sports 10:94; 1979.

15. Gennarelli, T.A.; Segave, H.; Wald, U.; Thibault, L.E. Physiological response to angular acceleration of the head. In: Grossman, R.G.; Gildenberg, P.L., eds. Head injury: basic and clinical aspects. New York: Raven Press; 1982:29-140.

16. Peerless, S.J. Rewcastle, N.B. Shear injuries of the brain. Can. Med. Assoc. J. 96:577-582; 1967.

17. Strich, S.J. Shearing of nerve fibers as a cause of brain damage due to head injury. Lancet 2:443-448; 1961.

18. Gurdjian, E.S.; Webster, J.E.; Lissner, H.R. Mechanism of skull fracture. Radiology 54:313; 1958.

19. Gronwall, D.; Wrightson, P. Delayed recovery of intellectual function after minor head injury. Lancet 2:605-609; 1974.

20. Gronwall, D. Paced auditory serial-addition task: a measure of recovery from concussion. Percept. Mot. Skills 44:367-373; 1977.

21. Gronwall, D.; Wrightson, P. Duration of post-traumatic amnesia after mild head injury. J. Clin. Neuropsychol. 2:51-60; 1980.

22. Gronwall, D.; Wrightson, P. Memory and information processing capacity after closed head injury. J. Neurol. Neurosurg. Psychiatry 44:889-895; 1981.

23. Schneider, R.C. Head and neck injuries in football: mechanisms, treatment, and prevention. Baltimore: Williams & Wilkins; 1973.

24. Saunders, R.L.; Harbaugh, R.E. The second impact in catastrophic contact-sports head trauma. JAMA 252:538-539; 1984.

25. Cantu, R.C. Guidelines for return to contact sports after cerebral concussion. Phy. Sportsmed. 14:75-83; 1986.

26. Kelley, J.P.; Nichols, J.S.; Filley, C.M.; Lillehei, K.O.; Rubinstein, D.; Kleinschmidt-DeMasters, B.K. Concussion in sports: guidelines for the prevention of catastrophic outcome. JAMA 266:2867-2869; 1991.

27. Martland, H.S. Punch drunk. JAMA 91:1103-1107; 1928.

28. Critchley, M. Medical aspects of boxing, particularly from a neurological standpoint. Br. Med. J. 1:357-362; 1957.

29. Busse, E.W.; Silvermen, A.J. Electroencephalographic changes in professional boxers. JAMA 149:1522-1525; 1952.

30. Kaplan, A.J.; Browder, J. Observations of the clinical and brain wave patterns of professional boxers. JAMA 156:1138-1144; 1954.

31. Betti, C.O.; Ottino, C.A. Pugilistic encephalopathy. Acta Neurol. Latino Americana 15:47-51; 1969.

32. Blonstein, J.L.; Clarke, E. Further observations on the medical aspects of amateur boxing. Br. Med. J. 1:362-364; 1957.

33. Brayne, C.E.G.; Dow, L.; Calloway, S.P.; Thompson, R.J. Blood creatinine kinase isoensyme BB in boxers. Lancet 2:1308-1309; 1982.

34. Brennan, T.N.N.; O'Connor, P.J. Incidence of boxing injuries in the Royal Air Force in the United Kingdom, 1953-1966. Br. J. Industr. Med. 25:326-329; 1968.

35. Colmant, H.J.; Dotzauer, G. Analyse eines todlich ausegangenen Boxkampfes mit ungewohnlich schweren cerebralen Schaden. Rechtsmedizin 84:263-278; 1980.

36. Courville, C.B. The mechanism of boxing fatalities. Bull. Los Angeles Neurol. Soc. 29:59-69; 1964.

37. Govons, S.R. Brain concussion and posture, the knockdown blow of the boxing ring. Confinia Neurologica 30:77-84; 1968.

38. Jedlinksi, J.; Gatarski, J.; Szymusik, A. Chronic posttraumatic changes in the central nervous system in pugilists. Pol. Med. J. 9:743-752; 1970.

39. Jedlinksi, J.; Gatarski, J.; Szymusik, A. Encephalopathia pugilistica (punch drunkenness). Acta Medica Pol. 12:443-451; 1971.

40. Johnson, J. Organic psych-syndrome due to boxing. Br. J. Psychiatry 115:45-53; 1969.

41. Kaste, M.; Vilkii, J.; Sainio, K.; Kuurne, T.; Katevuo, K.; Meurala, H. Is chronic brain damage in boxing a hazard of the past? Lancet 2:1186-1188; 1982.

42. Khosla, T.; Hitchens, R.A.N. Johnny Owen's ill-fated fight. Lancet 2:1254-1255; 1980.

43. Mawdsley, C.; Ferguson, F.R. Neurological disease in boxers. Lancet 2:795-801; 1963.

44. Paul, M. A fatal injury at boxing (traumatic decerebrate rigidity). Br. Med. J. 1:364-366; 1957.

45. Payne, E.E. Brains of boxers. Neurochirurgia 11:173-188; 1968.

46. Spillane, J.D. Five boxers. Br. Med. J. 2:1205-1210; 1962.

47. Roberts, A.H. Brain damage in boxers. London: Pitman; 1969:61-99.

48. Unterharnscheidt, F. About boxing: review of historical and medical aspects. Texas Reports on Biol. and Med. 28:421-495; 1970.

49. Corsellis, J.; Bruton, C.J.; Freeman-Browne, D. The aftermath of boxing. Psychol. Med. 3:270-303; 1973.

50. Ross, R.J.; Cole, M.; Thompson, J.S.; Kim, K.H. Boxers—computed tomography, EEG and neurological evaluation. JAMA 249:211-213; 1983.
51. Casson, I.R.; Sham, R.; Campbell, E.A., et al. Neurological and CT evaluation of knocked-out boxers. J. Neuro. Neurosurg. Psychiatry 45:170-174; 1982.

CHAPTER **4**

Amateur Boxing: Is There a Risk of Brain Injury?[†][*]

Walter F. Stewart
Barry Gordon

The risk of injury associated with boxing has been a long-standing medical and public health concern. In recent years, medical and professional societies have voiced their opposition to the sport (1-10) on the basis of observations of degenerative neurologic disorders resembling Parkinson's and Alzheimer's disease in professional boxers (11-13), reports of fatal injuries sustained during boxing matches, and ethical arguments against a sport in which injuring the opponent is perceived as the primary objective (6). Often in such discussions, no distinction is made between professional and amateur boxing. However, professional and amateur boxing differ in ways that may be important with respect to the motivation to compete

[†]This work was supported by the United States Olympic Foundation (1985-1988) and by NINCDS (NIH) Grant No. 26450 (1988-1995).

[*]This chapter was taken in part from "Prospective Study of Central Nervous System Function in Amateur Boxers in the United States" by W.F. Stewart, B. Gordon, O. Selnes, K. Bandeen-Roche, S. Zeger, R.J. Tusa, D.D. Celentano, A. Shechter, J. Liberman, C. Hall, D. Simon, R. Lesser, and R.D. Randall, 1994, *American Journal of Epidemiology*, **139**, pp. 573-588. Copyright 1994 by The Johns Hopkins University School of Hygiene and Public Health. Adapted by permission.

and the question of cerebral injury. (See chapter 2 for more on rule differences between amateur and pro boxing.) Moreover, while studies of professional boxers have indicated that there is a serious risk of brain damage, past studies of amateurs have been inconclusive.

In this chapter, we describe the rationale for and design and preliminary results of an ongoing, prospective study of amateur boxers (14). The primary objective of this study is to examine whether there is an excess risk of brain dysfunction from participation in amateur boxing as it is practiced today.

Review of Prior Studies

Amateur boxers have been examined in eight studies (Table 4.1) of the possible long-term risks of brain dysfunction or damage (15-22). The design of these studies varies considerably in terms of sample size, method of selecting amateur boxers, whether or not controls were used (and the type of control used), methods for medical assessment, and the criteria for defining abnormal/pathological status. Five of the studies had relatively large sample sizes and used controls (15-19), and four of these employed objective methods of neurological and neuropsychological assessment (16-19). The results of these studies are described next. Three studies (20-22) had design limitations considered too significant (including very small sample sizes, lack of a control group, and failure to use blind or objective methods of assessment) to allow one to make comparisons to other studies or to draw valid conclusions from the data. These studies are described in Table 4.1 for completeness, but are not examined in detail. Of the eight studies, the one by Haglund et al. (19) includes the most comprehensive set of measures. The results from neuropsychological testing are reviewed first, followed by a summary of results from other measures used.

Neuropsychological Assessment

Thomassen et al. (16) studied 53 former amateur boxers and 53 former soccer players. Fifty-three of 114 participants in the Denmark annual amateur boxing championships between 1955 and 1965 agreed to the study. Soccer players were matched on age and period of soccer career but not on level of education (the soccer players were significantly[1] better educated than the boxers). On each subject, the investigators completed a neurological exam, an EEG, and an extensive set of neuropsychologic measures. Overall, the boxers were significantly poorer on 5 of 30 neuropsychological measures (WAIS vocabulary, left hand motor function, repetitive speech, word synthesis, and logical memory). After adjusting for differences in education (analysis of a subset of boxers and soccer players matched on education), a statistically significant difference was found

Table 4.1 Summary of Studies of Amateur Boxers

Authors	Amateur boxers	Comparison group	Measures and findings and authors' conclusions	Study limitations
Jedlinski, Gatarski, & Szymusik (15)	60 active Polish boxers who competed before 1965 in 100 to 344 bouts	30 men "who wanted to take up boxing"	**Neurologic:** Signs in 55% of boxers, none in controls **Psychiatric:** Evidence of irritability, temper, psychomotor retardation, severe neuroses, psychoses, or character disorder in 18% of boxers and 0 controls **EEG:** Abnormal EEGs in 15% of boxers and 5% of controls <u>Authors' conclusions:</u> High level of impairment found in amateurs.	Multiple measures were used for boxers, single measures for controls. Assessments were not blind. Criteria for abnormal conditions were not established. Most measures were subjective. Reliability of the measures is questionable. Clinical significance of most signs, EEG disturbances, and psychomotor conditions appears to be minor.
Thomassen et al. (16)	53 former highly competitive Danish boxers who competed between 1955 and 1965 in 19 to 209 bouts	53 age-matched soccer players. Soccer players were better educated and held more skilled occupations.	**Neurologic:** No significant differences, but high prevalence of signs in boxers **Neuropsych:** After adjusting for education differences, boxers significantly poorer in left hand motor function ($p < .05$); consistently lower averages on some other measures but none significant **EEG:** No differences **Authors' conclusions:** Findings were inconclusive, especially after controlling for education.	Criteria for evaluating EEGs were not stated. Poor left hand motor function could be due to hand injuries common to boxers' nondominant hand.

(continued)

35

Table 4.1 (continued)

Authors	Amateur boxers	Comparison group	Measures and findings and authors' conclusions	Study limitations
Kaste et al. (20)	7 former and 1 active highly competitive Finnish boxer with an average of 129 bouts who competed in the 1960s and 1970s	Population norms	**Neurologic:** Normal **Neuropsych:** Normal except for trailmaking **EEG:** 4 of 7 "abnormal" **BEP:** 1 of 7 abnormal (lower amplitude on Wave V) **CT:** 1 of 8 with cavum septum pellucidum; 1 boxer with "abnormal" EEG, BEP, and CT <u>**Authors' conclusions:** Amateur boxing is associated with brain dysfunction.</u>	No control or comparison group was used. Criteria for defining "abnormal" were not well defined or adjusted for education and other factors.
Ross et al. (21)	11 former and 2 active U.S. boxers competing in 13 to 150 bouts; 9 former boxers competed before 1960.	None	**Neurologic:** 1 of 13 "abnormal" **EEG:** 4 of 8 "abnormal" **CT:** 5 of 13 "abnormal" <u>**Authors' conclusions:** Boxing causes brain damage.</u>	Representativeness of boxers is unknown. No information was given on antecedent factors. No explicit criteria were given for significant signs or EEG disturbances; no age criteria were given for abnormal CTs. No comparison population was used.

Study	Comparison group	Boxer population	Results	Comments
Casson et al. (22)	None	2 former and 3 active U.S. boxers. Former boxers competed in 1950s and 1960s. Boxers competed in 0 to 80 bouts.	**Neurologic:** 3 active boxers normal; 1 of 2 inactive boxers grossly abnormal **Neuropsych:** 3 active boxers "abnormal" on 2 of 8 tests; both former boxers "abnormal" on 5 of 8 tests **EEG and CT:** Active boxers "normal"; 1 of 2 former boxers grossly abnormal **Authors' conclusions:** Amateur boxing causes mild brain dysfunction.	Representativeness of boxers is unknown. No comparison population was used. No data on antecedents. No explicit criteria for significant signs, EEG disturbances, abnormal CTs, or abnormal neuropsych tests were given.
Brooks et al. (17)	19 men of comparable age, education, ethnicity	29 active British boxers who competed since the 1970s in 1 to 63 bouts	**Neuropsych:** 10 tests and 24 measures. Boxers significantly better on 1 (Progressive Matrices); controls significantly better on 2; on average, boxers were higher on 12 measures and controls on 6 **Authors' conclusions:** No consistent deficit in boxers and no association with boxing exposure were found.	Study had low statistical power. It may be too early to detect an effect.
McLatchie et al. (18)	Orthopedic patients and university students and staff of similar age	20 active Scottish boxers who competed in the 1970s and 1980s in 4 to 200 bouts	**Neurologic:** Significant abnormal signs in 2 to 4 of 20; 9 of 20 scored poorly on 2 measures, 3 of 20 scored poorly on all measures; boxers scored significantly poorer on Inglis Word Learning and Rey Figure **EEG:** Significant disturbances in 3 of 20 **CT:** Normal in 19 of 20 **Authors' conclusions:** A possible neuropsychological effect from boxing may exist.	Comparison populations may differ by education. Sample size is small, limiting study's statistical power. Abnormal clinical electrophysiological and neurological findings were excessively prevalent; the excess is not necessarily attributable to boxing.

(continued)

Table 4.1 (*continued*)

Authors	Amateur boxers	Comparison group	Measures and findings and authors' conclusions	Study limitations
Haglund et al. (19)	25 former Swedish amateur boxers with > 30 bouts; 25 former Swedish amateur boxers with < 10 bouts	25 soccer players and 25 track and field athletes	**Neurologic:** No differences **Psychologic:** Normal range of values **Neuropsych:** High-exposed boxers (> 30) had poorer finger tapping scores; no other differences **EEG:** No severe abnormalities; however, deviations in a higher proportion of boxers **P300:** No differences **CT:** Normal width of ventricles; higher proportion of boxers with cavum septum pellucidum **MRI:** No pathologic finding or differences **Authors' conclusions:** Amateur boxing has no statistically significant effect.	Study has low statistical power. Comparability of the controls to the boxers on socioeconomic factors is questionable.

only for one test (left hand motor function), but boxers were consistently poorer on a number of other tests. There were no statistically significant associations between any of the 30 neuropsychological measures and length of career, number of bouts, or number of K.O.s.

The neuropsychological measures used by Thomassen et al. (16) to test cognitive function are not widely accepted or used for research purposes, and the results cannot readily be compared to those of other studies. In addition, Brooks et al. (17) suggest that subtle cognitive impairments may not be detectable with these tests. In contrast, both McLatchie et al. (18) and Brooks et al. (17) used the same or similar neuropsychological measures, ones that are widely used for research on head injury-related impairments; their results are summarized in Table 4.2 by cognitive function tested.

Brooks et al. (17) tested 29 active amateur boxers (out of 75 invited to participate in the study) and compared them to 19 controls matched for age, ethnicity, and education. All subjects were 15 to 27 years of age. Boxers had significantly poorer scores (Table 4.2) on the immediate and delayed recall of a short story presented auditorially (Wechsler Memory Scale for Logical Memory), while controls had poorer scores on the Raven's Standard Progressive Matrices (a nonverbal measure of intelligence [IQ]).

McLatchie et al. (18) examined 20 amateur boxers ranging in age from 18 to 49. The boxers were selected or volunteered for examination and were compared on neuropsychological measures to a matched group of orthopedic outpatients with limb fractures and to a separate group of university students and staff. Matching criteria were not stated. Subjects were excluded if there was known exposure to solvents, previous head injury, or heavy drinking. Compared to the orthopedic outpatients (Table 4.1), the boxers were significantly poorer on the Inglis Word Learning test (verbal learning and memory) and the copy (visuoconstruction) and immediate recall (short-term visual memory) of the Rey Figure tests, but not on the Wechsler Memory Word Learning test, story recall (verbal learning and memory), Digit Span, or on computer-administered measures of visual memory and detection of visual change. On a four-choice reaction test, the boxers had significantly faster movement times but significantly slower decision times than university students and staff of a similar age.

Haglund et al. (19) have conducted the most comprehensive cross-sectional study to date. In the study 50 former amateur boxers (25 with > 30 bouts; 25 with < 10 bouts) were compared to 25 track and field athletes and 25 soccer players who were identified as "headers." Haglund et al. administered six neuropsychological tests (synonyms, blocks, Trails A and B, finger tapping, Claeson-Dahl verbal learning and retention, and memory for designs). A statistically significant difference was found only for the finger tapping test. Boxers with more than 30 bouts had poorer scores on both the dominant and nondominant hand.

Table 4.2 Summary of Neuropsychological Test Results in Two Comparable Studies of Amateur Boxers

General category	Specific task	Brooks[a]		McLatchie
		t	p	p
Attention/ concentration	Digit Span (F+B)[b]	0.57	ns	ns
	PASAT (slow)	0.76	ns	
	PASAT (fast)	0.12	ns	
Motor speed	Movement times			>.95
	Movement time (simple reaction)	1.21	ns	
	Movement time (choice reaction)	−0.33	ns	
	Finger tapping—R hand	−0.20	ns	
	Finger tapping—L hand	0.30	ns	
	Synchronous tapping			
	R hand	0.40	ns	
	L hand	0.10	ns	
Reaction time (rt)	Simple rt		ns	
	Simple decision time	0.01	ns	
	4-choice decision	1.21	ns	
	4-choice rt			<.05
	Visual detection (computer)			ns
Verbal learning/ memory[c]	Incidental	0.19	ns	
	Intentional	−0.68	ns	
	Wechsler Memory Scale			
	-Logical immed. recall	−2.53	<.01	ns
	-Logical delayed recall	−2.60	<.01	ns
	-Paired assoc.— old	−0.01	ns	ns
	-Paired assoc.— new	1.76	ns	ns
	Inglis Word Learning			<.05
Visual memory[c]	Visual detection (computer)			ns
	Visual span	−1.38	ns	
	Rey immediate recall	0.54	ns	<.05
	Computer visual memory			ns
Visuoconstruction	Rey copy	1.27	ns	<.05
Intelligence	Vocabulary	−1.31		<.01
	Progressive Matrices	2.62	>.99	

Note. ns = not statistically significant.
[a] t-test for difference. A positive t-test score indicates that the group score of boxers was better than that of controls. [b] F+B is forward span score plus backward span score. [c] Although the t-test for difference between point estimates was not statistically significant for some of the tests of this cognitive function, the variance for scores among boxers was significantly greater than that for controls.

Other Measures

Seven studies collected EEG data (15, 16, 18, 19, 20, 21, 22) and five studies completed CT scans on boxers (18, 19, 20, 21, 22). Jedlinski et al. (15) conducted repeated neurologic, EEG, and psychiatric examinations over a 4-year period of 60 Polish active amateur boxers who competed in 100 or more bouts in the 1950s and 1960s. One significant finding in this study was that 15% of the boxers had EEG tracings with slow waves, spikes, and spike-wave complexes, in comparison to 5% among controls. However, this difference may have been influenced by the fact that the boxers were examined multiple times while controls were examined only once. Thus the opportunity for finding abnormal EEG tracings was higher for boxers than for controls. In addition, the examinations were not done blindly, and the source and comparability of the controls were not described.

Thomassen et al. (16) reported that there were no statistically significant differences in the prevalence of EEG disturbances between their amateur boxers and soccer players. The criteria for identifying EEG disturbances were not stated.

McLatchie et al. (18) completed both CT scans and EEGs on boxers, but not on controls. All but one of the boxers had normal CT scans for their age. Eight of 20 boxers had abnormal EEGs, including several with minor disturbances and disturbances generally associated with younger age. Three of the eight boxers had significant disturbances. Neither the EEG nor the CT scans in the study by McLatchie et al. were read blindly.

Haglund et al. (19) collected data on EEG, P300 evoked potentials, and CT and MRI scans. While a higher proportion of boxers had EEG deviations and CT findings of a cavum septum pellucidum, there was no evidence from these four measures of significant abnormalities overall, and there were no meaningful differences among the boxers and control groups.

Summary

The major conclusions of these studies appear to be in the area of cognitive assessment. In two comparable studies (17, 18), amateur boxers did not do as well as controls on several neuropsychological tests. Statistically significant differences were found in both studies on verbal learning and memory, although different measures were used. Consistent differences were not found for any other cognitive functions tested. One limitation of verbal learning and memory tests compared to other neurophysiological tests is that they can be culturally and socially dependent. Thus, statistical comparisons are likely to be sensitive to the comparability of the control group selected. In Haglund et al. (19), amateur boxers and soccer players did not differ on neuropsychological tests. The results of this study can be interpreted in one of several ways: Since amateur boxing has changed, this study of more recent boxers indicates that safety in the sport has improved; the study was underpowered and only relatively large differences would have been detectable; or both boxers and soccer players are at risk of brain damage.

Overall, the results are not completely consistent either within or between studies. The relatively small sample sizes in these studies preclude us from concluding that there is no consistent pattern of risk that might be apparent in a larger, better controlled study. On the other hand, even where differences have been found, it is not possible to determine whether the differences between amateur boxers and controls are due to possible biases inherent to each of the study designs or causally related to participation in amateur boxing, a point noted by Brooks et al. (17) in reference to their own study. No study showed an association between neuropsychological test scores or other measures and number of bouts, length of time as an amateur, or number of times knocked out.

A concern in all five of these studies is that they are cross-sectional. In comparing the amateur boxers to the controls, two assumptions are implied. The first is that prior to any involvement in the sport of amateur boxing, boxers are identical or similar to nonboxers on neuropsychological tests and electrophysiological and other outcome measures of interest. Another implicit assumption is that, in comparison to boxers, nonboxers have the same history of exposure to antecedent factors that could cause or predispose them to brain dysfunction and damage. Moreover, since effects on these measures are not etiologically specific, these dysfunctions could occur in the absence of boxing and be attributable to other causes.

Implications for Study Design

The nature of the blows experienced in amateur boxing has several design implications for any study of the risk of brain dysfunction. First, what variables should be measured? From studies of head injury in general and professional boxers in particular, a number of specific anatomic sites appear to be susceptible to injury. Decrements from the normal level of function at these sites can in theory be measured by specific neuropsychologic and laboratory indices, including measures of memory, brainstem evoked potentials (23), and balance. Injury may, however, also cause less specific or more diffuse damage, with less clearly associated dysfunctions. Therefore, any assessment for such injury should also include measures sensitive to dysfunction in general, so that disturbances in central nervous system (CNS) processing not yet individually measurable can be detected.

Second, the existence of an impairment and its incidence must be measured in reference to a defined and relevant norm. The occurrence of so-called abnormal findings in any population can be quite high.[2] It is, therefore, important for any testing to be able to determine whether an apparent impairment is a true one, and whether any true impairment is caused by the specific condition of concern. Together, these problems interact with the measurement properties of the test itself.

A third issue of importance for the design of such a study is that the impairments that might occur from head injury may also be attributable to other causes. The frequency of such causes is population specific and depends on the prevalence of such factors as developmental impairments, substance and alcohol use, head injury, nutritional deficiency, CNS infections, and, in general, a subject's status prior to participation in amateur boxing.

Fourth, it is difficult to predict a priori the magnitude of an effect from amateur boxing, if such an effect exists at all, simply because most exposure is subconcussive. We know very little about the consequences of repeated subconcussive blows.

These considerations suggest that testing must be comprehensive and sensitive, that boxers from a wide range of exposures must be evaluated, that the study population must be large, and that an appropriate comparison population must be selected to make a valid judgment as to the existence of deficits due to participation in amateur boxing. Ideally, controls should be identical to boxers in all respects pertaining to CNS impairment except that they do not box. Finally, boxers should be examined while they are active, before any apparent effect might be expected, and study participants should be examined prospectively. In addition, as noted earlier (Review of Prior Studies), in cross-sectional studies there are fundamental and unverifiable assumptions that must be made with regard to the boxers and the comparison population. An advantage of the prospective design is that these assumptions can be relaxed. The focus of interest in the prospective design is the change in a subject's measurement or test performance between two or more points in time. As a result, differences between boxers and controls in measurement or performance status at entry into the study are not important as long as these differences do not interact with the degree or nature of the change in performance over time. Even confounding caused by this type of interaction can be measured and adjusted for in properly designed prospective studies.

Johns Hopkins Medical Institutions (JHMI) Study

In response to the controversy over amateur boxing and in recognition of the limitations of previous research, we initiated a study to determine if there is a risk of brain dysfunction from amateur boxing as it is currently practiced. The study was specifically designed to avoid many of the pitfalls of previous investigations, especially the inherent problems of attempting to infer causal associations from cross-sectional data.

In April 1986, after concerns were raised by the AMA and other medical societies, the United States Olympic Foundation (USOF), at the request of the USA/Amateur Boxing Federation (ABF), approved and funded a proposal by the JHMI to initiate a prospective study of active amateur boxers. A Technical Advisory Committee (TAC) composed of 10 experts in relevant disciplines was assembled to critically review the initial study plan.

The study was designed to specifically determine whether changes in selected neuropsychologic, neurologic, and electrophysiologic measures between baseline and follow-up examinations are associated with the degree of training and competition in amateur boxing. The study is unique in that

1. it is prospective, that is, subjects were identified before any apparent morbidity;
2. the study population is large;
3. a representative sample of amateur boxers was selected;
4. data were collected on antecedent factors;
5. a thorough test battery was employed; and
6. the focus is on a longitudinal comparison of effects.

Selection and Recruitment of Boxers

Since the inception of the study we were interested in locating a diverse and representative sample of clubs and in identifying active boxers with a range of experience, skills, and styles of boxing. On this basis and on the basis of the results of a nationwide club survey we conducted in 1985, six cities were selected from which to recruit and enroll amateur boxers for the prospective study. The six sites selected were Washington, DC; Houston, TX; Lake Charles, LA; Cleveland, OH; St. Louis, MO; and New York, NY. These sites were selected because of the relatively large number of resident amateur boxers and because the clubs were diverse in terms of type (strictly amateur clubs vs. clubs with both professional and amateur boxers), stability, number of boxers, age range of boxers, and experience of the athletes. All active members of the USA/ABF between 13 and 21 years of age in the six cities were eligible for testing and invited to participate.

A 35-foot GMC bus was converted into a mobile clinic for the purpose of the study. In the baseline study, enrollment of subjects at each study site was preceded by a meeting with coaches and officials to discuss the study and to answer questions. A preliminary list of eligible boxers from each club was obtained from coaches. A local recruiter visited each club periodically to meet with boxers, discuss the study, conduct a brief interview to determine eligibility, and invite participation. Parental consent was obtained if the subject was less than 18 years of age.

Comparison Population

The choice of the comparison population is critical to answering the question of what level of impairment is expected in the absence of amateur boxing; it is also central to a valid assessment of whether the sport causes CNS impairment. A number of different control groups were considered in consultation with our external advisory committee. Other amateur athletes were not thought to be comparable to amateur boxers on a number of potentially critical variables:

1. Boxers more often come from disadvantaged backgrounds. The prevalence of other causes of brain dysfunction is likely to be higher than expected.
2. Amateur boxing is not a scholastic sport. Boxers are not required to meet educational standards to participate.
3. There were logistical problems both in recruiting other athletes and in assuring that data were collected blind to the subject's athletic status. For example, amateur boxers could easily be distinguished from football or basketball players simply by their morphology.

We concluded that the optimal controls would be the boxers themselves, that is, subjects who signed up with the USA/ABF but who had little or no experience in competition. These subjects, whom we labeled the *low-exposure* group, were from the same neighborhood as other boxers; were likely to have had similar exposures to other, known and unknown neurologic insults (drugs, infections, violence, lead exposure, etc.); and were of the same stature, age, and socioeconomic, developmental, and educational backgrounds. In addition, they were relatively easy to identify and locate.

One limitation of the low-exposure controls is that they may not be as skilled athletically or as motivated specifically toward athletics as the more experienced boxers. If these athletic or motivational factors are related to the outcome measures of interest (e.g., neuropsychological test scores), spurious differences could occur at the time of the first examination that are not related to a subject's participation in the sport. For example, low-exposure boxers may actually perform less well on certain visuomotor tasks than more experienced boxers. A correct interpretation of such a trend cannot be obtained from a single set of cross-sectional measures. Therefore, as we have noted previously, a prospective design is necessary.

Examination Protocol

The examination protocol was developed with three primary considerations:

1. It must address theoretical issues and empirical evidence relevant to the functions or structures most likely to be affected by head blows.

2. It must be able to accommodate competing demands of training, school, or work.
3. It must not be so time-consuming as to negatively affect a subject's willingness to return for follow-up testing.

The following four points were specifically considered in developing the final examination protocol.

1. Brain structures most likely to be affected. On the basis of prior studies of head injury and experimental evidence, as reviewed earlier, the following anatomical sites may be particularly susceptible to damage from blows incurred in amateur boxing: the temporal lobes, the inferior frontal lobes and frontal poles, and the lower diencephalon and upper brainstem. Therefore, electrophysiologic and neurologic measures were selected that are sensitive to or specifically measure damage in these areas (e.g., contusions to frontal polar regions or axonal tearing in the brainstem) and that have been shown to be sensitive in subjects with mild-to-moderate head injury. Specifically, these measures include the Brainstem Auditory Evoked Responses (BAERs), an ataxia battery, and EEG monitoring with frequency and voltage analysis. The BAERs are electrical responses generated by the brainstem auditory pathways that occur within 10 seconds of an acoustic response (27). Other evoked measures were considered but were thought to be less feasible or reliable in a mobile clinic setting, such as visual evoked potentials, or unacceptable for research purposes, such as somatosensory evoked potentials. We chose three tests from the Ataxia Battery of Fregly et al. (28): the repeated trials for the Sharpened Romberg, standing on a beam with eyes closed, and standing on a beam with eyes open. These tests are sensitive to damage to the labyrinth in the inner ear, the vestibular nerve, the vestibular nucleus, and projections through the brainstem and cerebellum. EEGs have often been used in studies of head injury where contusion injury is suspected. Quantitative frequency and voltage analysis are used to summarize the EEG data. The functions mediated by the susceptible anatomical sites noted here and other factors discussed next were considered in selecting neuropsychological tests.

2. Test sensitivity and comparability. Results from published studies of professional boxers indicate the occurrence of mental and motor slowness, loss of concentration and memory, impaired and inappropriate judgment and actions, and other features of dementia (12, 28, 29). Furthermore, as noted in the review of previous studies, amateur boxers had lower average scores on a number of neuropsychological tests (17, 18). We considered such previously used tasks for inclusion, regardless of any specific questions about their interpretation, both because these tests appeared to be sensitive and because they would ensure that our results could be compared to those in the literature.

3. **Deficits underlying performance impairment.** The literature on concussion and mild-to-moderate closed head injury has suggested that deficits in attention and concentration, in new learning, and in retrieval from long-term memory underlie the performance impairments of such patients (30). Both the specific neuropsychological tasks already used and tasks reflecting these information-processing categories were considered.

4. **Technical constraints.** Technical constraints on the neuropsychological testing included commensurability across the 13 to 21-year age range, a wide dynamic range, relative insensitivity to education, reliability, previous standardization and experience (if possible), and ease of test taking. To maintain subject compliance, our pretest experience indicated that it was necessary to limit the total examination time to approximately four hours.

The optimal design, balancing scientific and practical issues, required maximizing the number of subjects enrolled, minimizing redundancies in the test protocol, and reducing the number of tests administered to each subject. The tests and measures used and other data collected during the baseline visit are described in Table 4.3. In addition to the electrophysiological and neurological measures described earlier, we selected a neuropsychological test battery to examine general intellectual functioning, attention and concentration, mental and motor speed, visuoconstruction, memory, and mental control and planning.

We did not employ structural measures such as CT or MRI for several reasons. Deficits in function are more significant and more meaningful than structural lesions that may or may not have behavioral significance. Also, neuropsychologic and neurophysiologic measures have been more sensitive than structural measures such as CT and MRI scans in reported studies of professional boxers (31) and studies of closed head injury (32). While this may change with improvements in technique, we did not feel it was appropriate to include these measures on such a large scale. For these reasons and for cost, safety, and feasibility considerations we ruled out CT/MRI scanning in the large group and other measures for ataxia/vestibular abnormalities, including caloric examination, head position-induced nystagmus, quantification of the vestibular ocular reflex by rotation in a chair, measurement of extraoculography, and quantitative posturography.

Sparring and Competition

Sparring is full-contact practice for competition, typically under the supervision of a coach and usually with a boxer comparable in size and skill. Competition refers to a bout sanctioned by USA Boxing. Exposure measures were derived separately for sparring and competition and defined separately for the period up to the baseline visit (X_1 in Figure 4.1) and

Table 4.3   Summary of Tests and Measures Used in the JHMI Prospective Study of Amateur Boxers

Type of data	Specific measure
Neuropsychologic tests	Raven's Progressive Matrices
	Digit Span, Forward
	Digit Span, Backward
	Rey Auditory Verbal Learning Test—Trial 1
	Symbol Digit Modalities test
	Computerized Vigilance test
	Grooved Pegboard
	2-Choice Reaction Time
	Finger Tapping test
	Block Design test (WAIS-R)
	Rey Complex Figure, Copy
	Rey Complex Figure, Immediate Recall
	Rey Auditory Verbal Learning Test
	Rey Complex Figure, Delayed Recall
	Trailmaking test
	Word Fluency Test (F,A,S)
Ataxia	Sharpened Romberg
	Standing on beam, eyes open
	Standing on beam, eyes closed
Electrophysiology	Brainstem Auditory Evoked Responses
	Electroencephalogram (EEG/CSA)
Interview	General health history
	Family profile
	Head injury history
	Education history
	Boxing history
	Substance use
	Psychosocial assessment
Substance use	Urine specimen
Physical	Dual neck measurements (top and base)

for the two-year interval between the baseline and follow-up examinations ($X_2 - X_1$ in Figure 4.1). Details regarding the interpretation of these measures are described elsewhere (14). Separate measures were defined for the period before the baseline examination and for the time period between the baseline and follow-up examinations. Exposure was defined in this manner so that bouts and sparring experience incurred during the follow-up interval could only affect test scores and other measures

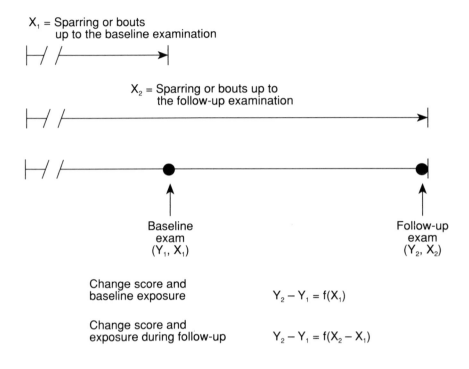

X_1 = Sparring or bouts
up to the baseline examination

X_2 = Sparring or bouts up to
the follow-up examination

Baseline
exam
(Y_1, X_1)

Follow-up
exam
(Y_2, X_2)

Change score and
baseline exposure

$$Y_2 - Y_1 = f(X_1)$$

Change score and
exposure during follow-up

$$Y_2 - Y_1 = f(X_2 - X_1)$$

Figure 4.1   Description of the relationships examined between outcome measures and sparring or bouts.

From "Prospective Study of Central Nervous System Function in Amateur Boxers in the United States" by W.F. Stewart et al., 1994, *American Journal of Epidemiology*, **139**, p. 577. Copyright 1994 by The Johns Hopkins University School of Hygiene and Public Health. Reprinted by permission.

obtained at follow-up. In contrast, bouts incurred before the baseline examination could have an effect on both the baseline and follow-up measures.

Sparring was defined as cumulative sparring-years and derived from reported data on sparring frequency and duration of sparring in years. For example, five sparring-years would be equal to sparring one 9-minute session per week for five years or sparring five 9-minute sessions per week for one year. Boxers were also defined as having never or ever sparred with a professional boxer. Knockouts in sparring or competition were too infrequent to be independently examined as exposure measures.

Statistical Methods

The outcome variable of interest was the change in cognitive, electrophysi- ologic, and neurologic measures over a two-year period (denoted as "change score"). The change score was separately analyzed as a categorical (i.e., subnormal vs. normal change) and continuous variable (using regression methods for longitudinal data to estimate mean change by exposure status). Moreover, analyses were completed in which the outcome was defined as the change score for an individual test and in which the outcomes were defined by the change score for a composite of tests for a specific functional domain (e.g., attention/concentration). In this chapter, we present detailed results for the analysis in which the outcome was defined as a categorical change variable (i.e., subnormal vs. normal change) for each of nine functional domains (Table 4.4). To describe change in the outcome measures, individuals were divided into two groups for each test or functional domain. If an individual's adjusted change score (14) was below the 16th percentile, he was arbitrarily defined as having subnormal change compared to all other subjects (see Figure 4.2). The conclusions based on the other methods of analysis described earlier were essentially the same as those described below in the results. Details regarding the method of selecting and summarizing measures for each functional domain and the statistical methods for analysis of data are presented elsewhere (14).

For each functional domain, logistic regression was used to compare subjects with subnormal change scores to all other subjects with regard to number of bouts and amount of sparring. The odds ratio was derived as a measure of association between the categorical change score (subnormal vs. normal change) and exposure variables. As an example of its interpretation, an odds ratio of 2.0 means that exposed individuals are twice as likely to have subnormal change scores as are nonexposed individuals.

Four separate exposure variables were defined as follows: number of bouts (0, 1-10, 11+) up to the baseline examination, number of bouts incurred during the follow-up interval, sparring-years (0, >0 to <5, 5+) up to the baseline examination, and sparring-years incurred during the follow-up interval. Before data analysis was initiated, the group boundaries for exposed subjects were selected as a balance between having an adequate number of individuals in each exposure group to estimate regression coefficients and limiting the range of values within a category. Ten bouts is also the maximum within the novice class. The odds ratios for number of bouts up to the baseline examination and during the follow-up intervals were estimated in the same model. Sparring-years was examined in a separate logistic regression model. The reference or zero-exposure category for estimating the odds ratio was specific to the bout or sparring variable of interest. For example, if a subject had no bouts up to the baseline examination and 15 bouts during the follow-up interval, he was placed in the zero-bout category for baseline exposure and in the highest bout category (i.e., 11+) for interval exposure.

Table 4.4 Functional Domains and Associated Tests and Measures*

Functional domains	Tests/Measures
Perceptual/motor	Blocks Design Symbol Digit Trailmaking Test B
Attention/concentration	Digit Span, Forward Digit Span, Backward Rey Auditory Verbal Learning Test—Trial 1 Symbol Digit Vigilance D′ (accuracy)
Psychomotor speed	Average of Grooved Pegboard for right and left hand Trailmaking Test A Trialmaking Test B
Memory	Rey Auditory Verbal Learning Test—Trial 5 Rey Complex Figure, Immediate Recall Rey Complex Figure, Delayed Recall
Visuoconstruction	Blocks Design Rey Complex Figure, Copy
Mental control	Trailmaking Test A Trailmaking Test B Word Fluency Test (F,A,S) Digit Span, Forward Digit Span, Backward
Ataxia	Sharpened Romberg Standing on beam, eyes open Standing on beam, eyes closed
Brainstem Auditory Evoked Responses (BAERs)	Wave I-V midlatency, left ear Wave I-V midlatency, right ear Amplitude ratio (Wave I/Wave V) left ear, right ear
EEG	Compressed Spectral Array average alpha frequency, left ear Compressed Spectral Array average alpha frequency, right ear Compressed Spectral Array alpha frequency, difference

*From "Prospective Study of Central Nervous System Function in Amateur Boxers in the United States" by W.F. Stewart et al., 1994, *American Journal of Epidemiology*, **139**, p. 578. Copyright 1994 by The Johns Hopkins University School of Hygiene and Public Health. Reprinted by permission.

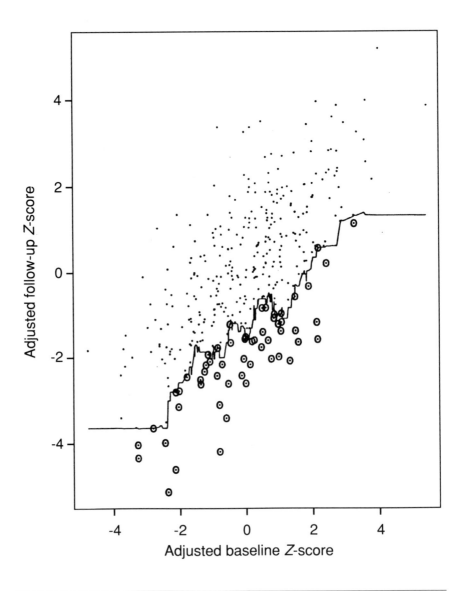

Figure 4.2 Distribution of subjects by adjusted Z-score at baseline and follow-up for the perceptual/motor domain (circled dots identify subjects with subnormal change scores, i.e., ≤ 16th percentile).

From "Prospective Study of Central Nervous System Function in Amateur Boxers in the United States" by W.F. Stewart et al., 1994, *American Journal of Epidemiology*, **139**, p. 579. Copyright 1994 by The Johns Hopkins University School of Hygiene and Public Health. Reprinted by permission.

Of the 393 boxers examined at follow-up, 24 had boxed one or more professional bouts since their baseline examination and were, therefore, excluded from the current analysis, leaving 369 participants for the prospective analysis. Four additional subjects were excluded from the analysis because data from the baseline or follow-up ($n=2$) visits were incomplete or because boxing histories reported at baseline and follow-up were highly discrepant and could not be resolved ($n=2$).

Results

The following are the results of the study, including a description of the population studied and an analysis of the data collected.

Population Description

Forty-three percent of the amateur boxers enrolled at baseline were 13 to 15 years of age; 50% were African-American (Table 4.5) (14), and 25% were Hispanic and primarily from New York City (48.5% Hispanic) and Houston (67.1% Hispanic). In general, educational achievement was low, but at the expected level given that most subjects resided in inner-city areas. Twenty-seven percent of the boxers were at least one grade behind in school for their age, and 11% of those 18 years and older had not finished high school. Reported concussive head injury from causes external to boxing was common; approximately 12% reported at least one concussive head injury with unconsciousness not due to boxing. The two most common causes were bicycle accidents and being hit by a club or bat. Among those who completed both the baseline and follow-up examinations, 7.9% had a positive urine drug test at baseline, 15.6% tested positive at follow-up, and overall, 4.7% tested positive at both examinations. The urine drug test was sensitive to drugs used in the previous one to two weeks. Marijuana was the most common finding on positive tests.

Exposure-Response Analysis

For each functional domain, the odds ratio was estimated as a measure of association between change score status (subnormal vs. normal) and bout group (0, 1-10, and 11+). Again, as an example of its interpretation, an odds ratio of 2.0 for subjects boxing 11 or more bouts up to the baseline examination means that a subject who boxed 11 or more bouts before the baseline examination is twice as likely to have subnormal change scores as nonexposed individuals. Odds ratios were separately estimated for bouts incurred up to the baseline visit (Table 4.6, upper panel, page 56) and for bouts incurred between the baseline and follow-up visits (Table 4.6, lower panel, page 57). Odds ratios were estimated for sparring-years in a similar manner (Table 4.7, pages 58-59).

Table 4.5 **Percent Distribution of Study Subjects at Baseline and Follow-up by Selected Variables Measured During the Baseline Examinations***

Variable	Category	Baseline examination ($n = 456$) %	Follow-up examination ($n = 365$) %
Site	Washington	12.9	12.6
	Houston	14.0	12.6
	Louisiana	10.5	11.8
	Cleveland	12.3	12.1
	St. Louis	24.1	25.2
	New York	26.1	25.8
Age at baseline	13-15	43.4	45.2
	16-17	30.1	30.4
	18+	26.5	24.4
Race	Black	50.9	52.3
	Hispanic	24.6	24.4
	White	24.6	23.3
Highest education	≤ 8th grade	47.8	45.8
	9th-11th grade	39.9	42.5
	12th grade +	12.3	11.8
Behind in school for age	No	72.1	73.2
	Yes	27.9	26.8
Father's education	<High school	22.6.	22.7
	High school	29.2	28.5
	>High school	17.8	18.4
	Do not know	30.5	30.4
Mother's education	<High school	27.6	27.1
	High school	33.6	33.7
	>High school	17.8	18.9
	Do not know	21.1	20.3
Reported concussion	0	87.5	87.1
	1+	12.5	12.8
Urine test[a]	−	79.4	80.5
	+	7.9	7.7
	r	1.8	0.8
	NA	11.0	11.0

[a]Results of urine drug test at baseline and follow-up are denoted as negative (−), positive (+), refused (r), or not applicable (NA).

*From "Prospective Study of Central Nervous System Function in Amateur Boxers in the United States" by W.F. Stewart et al., 1994, *American Journal of Epidemiology*, **139**, p. 580. Copyright 1994 by The Johns Hopkins University School of Hygiene and Public Health. Reprinted by permission.

Competitive Bouts: At the age of their first bout, 15% of the participants were 10 years of age or less and 45% were 11 to 15 years of age. At enrollment, 29% of the subjects had been competing for five or more years. Moreover, at baseline, 13% of subjects had had a bout within two weeks of their visit; 7% of the participants had a bout within two weeks of their follow-up examination. However, the time interval between testing and the last bout was not associated with test scores (14).

No statistically significant odds ratios were found for the association between change score status and bouts incurred up to the baseline visit (Table 4.6, upper panel, page 56) (14). However, statistically significant tests of linear trend were found for the memory, perceptual/motor, and visuoconstruction domains. The blocks test, a timed measure of visuoconstructional abilities, was common to the latter two domains. It is noteworthy that before initiating the study, we predicted that memory function was likely to decline due to brain damage. However, we did not predict that visuoconstructional or perceptual/motor abilities would decline in the early stages of progressive brain damage (14).

In contrast to bouts incurred before baseline, no statistically significant tests of trend or elevated odds ratios were found for the association between change score (subnormal vs. normal) and number of bouts incurred during the follow-up interval (Table 4.6, lower panel, page 57). These results are consistent with the analysis of individual tests.

Sparring: Virtually all boxers wore headgear during sparring, but sparring practice itself varied considerably between boxers. Ninety-five percent of sparring sessions ranged from 2 to 18 minutes (rounds × minutes per round) in length, varying either because the duration of rounds (from 1 to 4 minutes) or the number of rounds per sparring session (1 to 7) varied. As of the baseline visit, 20% of the study participants had never sparred, 69% had been sparring for 12 months or more, and 48% had been sparring for two years or more. During the follow-up interval, 18% of the boxers did not spar; 49% had sparred for 18 to 24 months of the two-year period. Six boxers at baseline and 12 at follow-up reported being knocked out during sparring.

Overall, no statistically significant associations emerged from the analysis of sparring-years (Table 4.7, pages 58-59). Nonetheless, in several respects, the pattern of associations for sparring up to baseline is similar to that found for bouts. Elevated but nonsignificant odds ratios were found for memory, perceptual/motor abilities, and visuoconstructional abilities with sparring up to baseline, the same domains for which significant tests of trend were found with number of bouts up to baseline. When bouts up to baseline was added to the model, the odds ratio for the highest sparring-years group (5+ sparring-years), but not the middle group, declined (14).

For sparring-years during the follow-up interval (Table 4.7, lower panel, page 59), again no statistically significant odds ratios or tests of trend

Table 4.6 Odds Ratios for the Association Between Change Score (Subnormal vs. Normal) and Bout Group[a] at Baseline and During the Follow-Up Interval by Each of Nine Functional Domains*

Test domain	Change score status	Subjects by bout group			Odds ratio (95% CI) by bout groups	
		0	1-10	11+	1-10	11+
					Bouts incurred up to baseline	
Perceptual/motor	Subnormal	8	18	30	1.22 (0.50, 3.01)	2.21 (0.89, 5.43)[b]
	Normal	72	127	109		
Attention/concentration	Subnormal	13	24	21	0.94 (0.44, 2.01)	0.67 (0.29, 1.56)
	Normal	67	121	118		
Psychomotor speed	Subnormal	13	20	22	0.90 (0.41, 1.96)	1.21 (0.53, 2.75)
	Normal	66	125	116		
Memory	Subnormal	9	19	31	1.23 (0.52, 2.92)	2.23 (0.94, 5.27)[b]
	Normal	71	126	108		
Visuoconstruction	Subnormal	11	17	31	0.91 (0.40, 2.08)	2.20 (0.97, 5.02)[b]
	Normal	70	127	107		
Mental control	Subnormal	16	22	22	0.72 (0.34, 1.51)	0.66 (0.30, 1.45)
	Normal	64	123	117		
Ataxia	Subnormal	12	18	20	0.75 (0.33, 1.70)	1.12 (0.47, 2.62)
	Normal	52	110	93		
BAERs	Subnormal	9	24	21	1.46 (0.63, 3.40)	1.16 (0.47, 2.86)
	Normal	62	104	104		
EEG	Subnormal	15	17	20	0.56 (0.26, 1.23)	0.82 (0.36, 1.86)
	Normal	53	116	106		

					Bouts incurred during the follow-up interval	
Perceptual/motor	Subnormal	9	18	29	0.98 (0.41, 2.33)	1.26 (0.53, 2.98)
	Normal	63	123	122		
Attention/concentration	Subnormal	12	15	31	0.61 (0.27, 1.38)	1.50 (0.67, 3.33)
	Normal	60	126	120		
Psychomotor speed	Subnormal	13	23	19	0.86 (0.40, 1.85)	0.58 (0.26, 1.33)
	Normal	57	118	132		
Memory	Subnormal	12	18	29	0.70 (0.31, 1.56)	0.89 (0.40, 2.00)
	Normal	60	123	122		
Visuoconstruction	Subnormal	12	23	24	0.98 (0.45, 2.15)	0.69 (0.30, 1.57)
	Normal	60	117	127		
Mental control	Subnormal	15	17	28	0.55 (0.26, 1.18)	1.01 (0.47, 2.16)
	Normal	57	124	123		
Ataxia	Subnormal	10	23	17	1.16 (0.51, 2.65)	0.76 (0.30, 1.90)
	Normal	49	101	105		
BAERs	Subnormal	8	19	27	1.12 (0.45, 2.75)	1.52 (0.62, 3.75)
	Normal	53	105	112		
EEG	Subnormal	12	22	18	0.94 (0.42, 2.09)	0.64 (0.27, 1.51)
	Normal	48	105	122		

[a]Baseline and interval terms in the same model. [b]$p < 0.05$ for trend test.

*From "Prospective Study of Central Nervous System Function in Amateur Boxers in the United States" by W.F. Stewart et al., 1994, *American Journal of Epidemiology*, **139**, pp. 582-583. Copyright 1994 by The Johns Hopkins University School of Hygiene and Public Health. Reprinted by permission.

Table 4.7 Odds Ratios for the Association Between Change Score (Subnormal vs. Normal) and Sparring-Years Group[a] at Baseline and During the Follow-Up Interval by Each of Nine Functional Domains*

Test domain	Change score status	Subjects by sparring group			Odds ratio (95% CI) by sparring groups	
		0	>0, <5	5+	>0, <5	5+
					Sparring up to baseline	
Perceptual/motor	Subnormal	6	23	27	1.72 (0.63, 4.66)	1.91 (0.69, 5.31)
	Normal	63	123	122		
Attention/concentration	Subnormal	13	30	15	1.22 (0.56, 2.68)	0.53 (0.22, 1.27)
	Normal	56	116	134		
Psychomotor speed	Subnormal	9	21	25	0.98 (0.40, 2.41)	1.26 (0.51, 3.10)
	Normal	60	125	122		
Memory	Subnormal	6	26	27	2.62 (0.96, 7.10)	2.57 (0.93, 7.16)
	Normal	63	120	122		
Visuoconstruction	Subnormal	7	28	24	1.98 (0.77, 5.06)	1.58 (0.61, 4.14)
	Normal	60	119	125		
Mental control	Subnormal	10	23	27	0.86 (0.36, 2.04)	0.97 (0.41, 2.29)
	Normal	59	123	122		
Ataxia	Subnormal	9	25	16	0.92 (0.38, 2.23)	0.55 (0.22, 1.42)
	Normal	37	106	112		
BAERs	Subnormal	12	17	25	0.54 (0.23, 1.29)	0.96 (0.41, 2.23)
	Normal	47	118	105		
EEG	Subnormal	15	16	21	0.37 (0.16, 0.88)[b]	0.44 (0.18, 1.03)
	Normal	45	116	114		

				Sparring during the follow-up interval	
Perceptual/motor	Subnormal	7	27	22	1.18 (0.46, 3.04)	1.66 (0.63, 4.44)
	Normal	60	161	87		
Attention/concentration	Subnormal	13	30	15	0.81 (0.37, 1.78)	0.80 (0.33, 1.98)
	Normal	54	158	94		
Psychomotor speed	Subnormal	7	33	15	1.70 (0.68, 4.27)	1.21 (0.43, 3.42)
	Normal	58	155	94		
Memory	Subnormal	11	27	21	0.62 (0.27, 1.42)	0.83 (0.34, 2.00)
	Normal	56	161	88		
Visuoconstruction	Subnormal	9	30	20	0.97 (0.42, 2.25)	1.12 (0.44, 2.80)
	Normal	56	158	90		
Mental control	Subnormal	7	31	22	1.76 (0.70, 4.44)	2.23 (0.82, 6.05)
	Normal	60	157	87		
Ataxia	Subnormal	7	29	14	1.19 (0.47, 3.07)	1.23 (0.43, 3.56)
	Normal	38	143	74		
BAERs	Subnormal	8	32	14	1.36 (0.54, 3.42)	0.90 (0.34, 2.41)
	Normal	42	141	87		
EEG	Subnormal	10	21	21	0.82 (0.34, 1.98)	1.72 (0.64, 4.57)
	Normal	42	152	81		

[a]Baseline and interval terms in the same model. [b] $p < 0.05$ for individual sparring category.

*From "Prospective Study of Central Nervous System Function in Amateur Boxers in the United States" by W.F. Stewart et al., 1994, *American Journal of Epidemiology*, **139**, pp. 584-585. Copyright 1994 by The Johns Hopkins University School of Hygiene and Public Health. Reprinted by permission.

were found for the association with subnormal change scores. Overall, these results are consistent with the results from the analysis of individual tests, where the number of significant findings was similar to that expected by chance.

Sparring With a Professional Boxer: A relatively large number of amateur boxers reported that they had sparred with a professional boxer on one or more occasions. However, frequent sparring with a professional was uncommon. To determine whether sparring with a professional was a risk factor for subnormal change scores, odds ratios were estimated by functional domain for infrequent and frequent sparring with a professional, adjusted for total number of sparring-years. Among nine functional domains, a marginally significant odds ratio ($p < 0.06$) was found only for attention/concentration and those who frequently sparred with a professional (odds ratio = 3.12). The odds ratio was 1.63 for boxers who sparred with a professional but did so infrequently. No other elevated odds ratios emerged from the analysis of this exposure variable.

Discussion

Before data analysis was initiated we expected that, if amateur boxing caused CNS damage, attention/concentration was the most likely function to be impaired, followed by visual/verbal memory and some forms of motor function. In our analysis, we found a statistically significant association between change in memory function and number of bouts up to baseline. No statistically significant associations were found with attention/concentration. In contrast, the statistically significant association between number of bouts up to baseline and perceptual/motor and visuoconstructional abilities was not expected. Elevated but nonsignificant odds ratios were found with sparring-years in these same domains. However, this last association appears to be due to the correlation between bouts and sparring-years.

It is noteworthy that significant associations were found only with number of bouts incurred up to the baseline visit and not for bouts incurred during the follow-up interval. There are several possible explanations for this finding. The behavioral consequences of head injury may be expressed only after a number of years. In our analysis, bouts up to baseline were incurred from 1 to more than 10 years before the baseline examination. In contrast, bouts taking place during the follow-up interval occurred within two years of the follow-up examination. Thus, duration of time since first exposure may be an important factor in determining when CNS effects are expressed or are detectable. As an alternative explanation, new safety measures implemented between 1984 and 1986 may account for the observed pattern of associations. Safety practice in amateur boxing was significantly modified between 1984 and 1986. Thus, the observed statistically significant odds ratios between selected cognitive domains and number of bouts up to baseline may reflect more severe exposure from single bouts during a time when safety regulations were less strict (i.e., before 1984). In the current data-set, it is not possible to determine which of these two factors provides the best explanation for the observed associations because there is a relatively strong correlation between duration of time since first bout and number of bouts before baseline. However, continued follow-up of this population will allow us to determine more directly whether time since first exposure is a meaningful explanatory variable or whether the observed effect is attributable to exposure incurred during a period when safety regulations were not as strict as they are today.

No statistically significant associations were found between sparring and any test domain. This was contrary to what we expected, because sparring sessions are considerably more common than competitive bouts. Several explanations may account for the absence of significant findings. First, exposure during sparring may not be severe enough to cause brain damage. Second, if exposure from sparring is less severe, a longer latency period may be required before impaired function is manifest. Finally, in contrast to number of bouts, sparring may be reported with greater error. As a result, the magnitude of the odds ratio will be underestimated and significant associations may not emerge.

We also estimated odds ratios between exposure (i.e., bouts and sparring-years) and individual tests. A total of 27 different measures were examined (54 odds ratios per exposure variable). Before analysis was initiated, we expected that the following tests would be the most sensitive to impairments (in declining order of sensitivity): vigilance, Trails B and Symbol Digit, and the Rey Complex Figure (Immediate and Delayed Recall) and the Rey Auditory Verbal Learning test (total score). We found no consistent evidence from this analysis of individual tests that met with our prior expectation.

In conclusion, this prospective study of a representative sample of amateur boxers provides supporting evidence that an increased number of bouts in the past is associated with diminished performance in selected cognitive domains. None of the changes we have observed to date, however, are clinically significant. Nonetheless, continued follow-up of this population will help explain whether the observed associations are transient or persistent, as well as whether a minimal latency period or more severe exposure in the past accounts for the observed associations and, if so, whether the changes are progressive.

Notes

[1]*Significantly* is used here to mean statistically significant.

²As an example, consider EEG slowing, which has often been used in studies of boxers and widely treated as pathologic. However, slowing is also known to be common at younger ages, declining with advancing age (24). Many EEG findings are transient and have little or no clinical significance (24). Up to 20% of the population has been reported to have "abnormal" tracings on a single exam (25). Moreover, the simple detection of EEG disturbances can be highly subjective and depends on a number of factors including the frequency of examinations, knowledge of the subject's status (e.g., head injured or not), and the precision with which disturbances are defined (26).

References

1. Council on Scientific Affairs. Brain injury in boxing. JAMA 249:254-257; 1983.
2. Hage, P. To ban or not to ban? Phy. Sportsmed. 11:143; 1983.
3. Lundberg, G.D. Boxing should be banned in civilized countries. JAMA 249:250; 1983.
4. Van Allen, M.W. The deadly degrading sport [editorial]. JAMA 249:250-251; 1983.
5. American Academy of Pediatrics Committee on Sports Medicine. Participation in boxing among children and young adults. Pediatrics 74:311-312; 1984.
6. Lundberg, G.D. Boxing should be banned in civilized countries—round 2. JAMA 251:2692-2698; 1984.
7. Ludwig, R. Making boxing safer: the Swedish model. JAMA 255:2482; 1986.
8. Lundberg, G.D. Boxing should be banned in civilized countries—round 3 [editorial]. JAMA 255:2483-2485; 1986.
9. Morrison, R.G. Medical and public health aspects of boxing. JAMA 255:2475-2480; 1986.
10. Patterson, R.H. On boxing and liberty. JAMA 255:2481-2482; 1986.
11. Roberts, A.H. Brain damage in boxers. London: Pittman Medical and Scientific Publishing; 1969.
12. Johnson, J. Organic psychosyndromes due to boxing. Br. J. Psychiatry 115:45-53; 1969.
13. Corsellis, J.A.; Bruton, C.J.; Freeman-Browne, D. Aftermath of boxing. Psychol. Med. 3:270-303; 1973.
14. Stewart, W.F.; Gordon, B.; Selnes, O.; Bandeen-Roche, K.; Zeger, S.; Tusa, R.J.; Celentano, D.D.; Shechter, A.; Liberman, J.; Hall, C.; Simon, D.; Lesser, R.; Randall, R.D. Prospective study of central nervous system function in amateur boxers in the United States. Am. J. Epidemiol. 139:573-588; 1994.
15. Jedlinski, J.; Gatarski, J.; Szymusik, A. Encephalopathia pugilistica (punch drunkeness) Acta Med. Pol. 12:443-451; 1970.

16. Thomassen, A.; Juul-Jensen, P.; Olivarius, B.; Braemer, J.; Christenson, A.L. Neurological, electroencephalographic and neuropsychological examination of 53 former amateur boxers. Acta Neurol. Scand. 60:352-362; 1979.

17. Brooks, N.; Kupshik, G.; Galbraith, S.; Ward, R. A neuropsychological study of active amateur boxers. J. Neurol. Neurosurg. Psychiatry 50:997-1000; 1987.

18. McLatchie, G.; Brooks, N.; Galbraith, S.; Hutshinson, J.S.F.; Wilson, L.; Melville, I.; Teasdale, E. Clinical neurological examination, neuropsychology, electroencephalography and computed tomographic head scanning in active amateur boxers. J. Neurol. Neurosurg. Psychiatry 50:96-99; 1987.

19. Haglund, Y.; Eriksson, E. Does amateur boxing lead to chronic brain damage? Am. J. Sports Med. 21:91-104; 1993.

20. Kaste, M.; Kuurne, T.; Vilkki, J.; Katevuo, K.; Sainio, K.; Meurala, H. Is chronic brain damage in boxing a hazard of the past? Lancet 2:1186-1188; 1982.

21. Ross, R.J.; Cole, M.; Thompson, J.S.; Kim, K.H. Boxers—computed tomography, EEG, and neurological evaluation. JAMA 249:211-213; 1983.

22. Casson, I.R.; Siegel, O.; Sham, R.; Campbell, E.A.; Tarlau, M.; DiDomenico, A. Brain damage in modern boxers. JAMA 251:2663-2667; 1984.

23. Gronwall, D.; Wrightson, P. Cumulative effect of concussion. Lancet 2:995-997; 1975.

24. Petersen, I., Feg-Olofosson, O. The development of the electroencephalogram in normal children from the age of one through fifteen years. Neuropaeditrie 2:247-304; 1971.

25. Sharbrough, F.W. Nonspecific abnormal EEG patterns. In: Niedermeyer, E.; Lopez de Silva, F., eds. Electroencephalography—basic principles, clinical applications, and related fields. Baltimore: Urban and Schwarzenberg; 1987: p. 163-181.

26. Niedermeyer, E. Abnormal EEG patterns. In: Niedermeyer, E.; Lopez de Silva, F., eds. Electroencephalography—basic principles, clinical applications, and related fields. Baltimore: Urban and Schwarzenberg; 1987: p. 183-208.

27. Schoenhuber, R.; Bortolotti, P.; Malavasi, P.; Marzolini, S.; Tonelli, L.; Merli, G.A. Brainstem auditory evoked potentials in early evaluation of cerebral concussion. J. Neurosurg. Sci. 27:157-159; 1983.

28. Fregley, A.R.; Smith, M.J.; Graybiel, A. Revised normative standards of performance of men on a quantitative ataxia test battery. Acta Otolaryngeal (Stockh) 75:10-16; 1973.

29. Martland, H.S. Punch drunk. JAMA 91:1103; 1928.

30. Gennarelli, T.A.; Adams, J.H.; Graham, D.I. Acceleration induced head injury in the monkey: I. The model, its mechanical and physiological correlates. Acta Neuropathol. VII:23-25; 1981.

31. Casson, I.R.; Sham, R.; Campbell, E.A.; Tarlau, M.; DiDomenico, A. Neurological and CT evaluation of knocked-out boxers. J. Neurol. Neurosurg. Psychiatry 45:170-174; 1982.
32. Cullum, C.M.; Bigler, E.D. Late effects of hematoma on brain morphology and memory in closed head injury. Int. J. Neurosci. 28:279-283; 1985.

CHAPTER 5

Eye Injuries

Vincent J. Giovinazzo

David J. Smith

Paul F. Vinger

Boxing is a preventable cause of blindness. Vision defects from boxing are due to the shock waves and compressive effects of blows to the eye(s) themselves, the periorbital and orbital bones and soft tissues, or the visual centers and pathways from the optic nerves to the occipital cortices.

In this chapter we will discuss the typical ocular and visual disabilities secondary to boxing, their incidence in amateur and professional boxing, and suggestions for reduction of permanent visual disability to boxers.

Eye and Visual Boxing Injuries

Eye and visual injuries that can be caused by boxing include injuries to the eye and its contents, to the central visual pathways, or to the periorbita and orbit.

Injuries to the Eye and Ocular Contents

Possible boxing injuries to the eye are a ruptured or perforated globe, hyphema, cataracts, retinal tears or detachment, and macula injuries.

Ruptured or Perforated Globe: Although thumbing (which transmits the greatest possible force to the globe) has resulted in one incident of a ruptured globe, a normal eye would usually not be perforated or ruptured by the blunt forces involved in the sport. However, a major concern is the strength of healed wounds to the cornea and sclera from surgery. Radial keratotomy (the surgical correction of myopia) weakens the cornea, as do incisions from prior cataract surgery. Since this structural weakness probably lasts for life, radial keratotomy is not recommended for boxers. Boxers who have had prior eye surgery of any type require close postfight observation by an ophthalmologist.

Hyphema: Hyphema, or bleeding into the anterior chamber, is common and is due to tearing of vessels at the iris root. Often associated with hyphema are pigment dispersion and recession and scarring (anterior synechiae) of the iridocorneal angle and the trabecular meshwork; these may result in glaucoma and loss of vision years after the injury. All boxers who have experienced hyphema need gonioscopy to evaluate the possibility of late onset glaucoma. Rubeosis iridis may also result in late glaucoma. Iris sphincter tears may cause pupillary irregularity.

Cataracts: This opacity of the lens resulting in decreased vision is common, most often posterior subcapsular in boxers (Figure 5.1), and is often treated by surgery to remove the opaque lens and insert a plastic intraocular lens implant. If the cataract is the only ocular defect present, surgery is usually successful. A return to boxing after cataract surgery should be discouraged because of uncertainty of the strength of the healed wounds and the stability of the intraocular lens with repeated blows to the eye. With small-incision cataract surgery, boxers have a better chance to return to the ring.

Retinal Tears and Detachment: Blows may cause either tears in the retina or a complete detachment. Although retinal tears and retinal detachments are undeniably linked, the difference in prognosis and severity justifies a separation. The state of California prohibits any boxer from obtaining a license if he has suffered a retinal detachment or a retinal tear. However, the authors believe that many boxers with successfully repaired retinal detachments may continue their careers and that a treated retinal tear should almost never compel a boxer to retire.

Rips, breaks, or tears in the retina occur when the globe is suddenly compressed and traction from the vitreous rips a tear in the retina. If blood vessels are also torn, vitreous hemorrhage may be present (which may obscure the tear). Retinal tears can also occur when direct trauma causes such extensive damage that necrotic holes develop in the retina. Retinal dialyses are seen in boxers when the retina separates at its most anterior extension, the ora serrata, from its attachment to the pars plana. Retinal tears, if untreated, will frequently progress to a retinal detachment. Treatment of retinal tears with either laser or cryotherapy will prevent their progression with virtually no side effects (Figure 5.2, page 68).

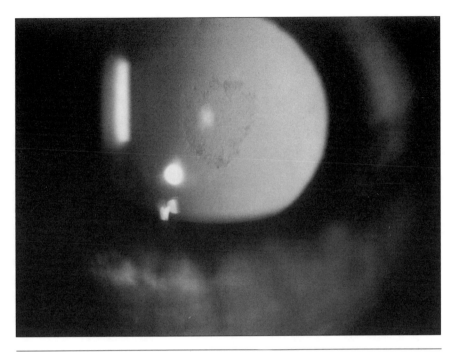

Figure 5.1 Posterior subcapsular cataract in a 19-year-old boxer.

Retinal detachment is caused by retinal tears and leaking of liquefied vitreous through the tear into the potential space between the retina and the retinal pigment epithelium (Figure 5.3, a-b, page 69). Large defects of the peripheral visual field may be present, as well as loss of central vision from detachment of the central retina, the macula. Surgical repair is usually successful, but vision may remain permanently impaired once the macula is detached or if there is coexisting retinal scarring. Retinal tears and detachments should be treated as early as possible to prevent permanent visual loss.

Macula Injuries: Compression of the globe can cause a rupture of the choroid and create an underlying scar that reduces central vision. Trauma may also cause intraretinal edema (commotio retinae). As a consequence of macula edema, a macula hole may develop, with loss of central vision. All macula injuries have the potential for a permanent reduction of central visual acuity. Since the retina is actually central nervous tissue, there is no hope of recovering vision lost to traumatic retinal scarring involving the macula.

Injuries to the Central Visual Pathways

The optic nerves, optic chiasm, optic tracts, and visual cortex are susceptible to permanent damage from repeated blows to the head. Cortical

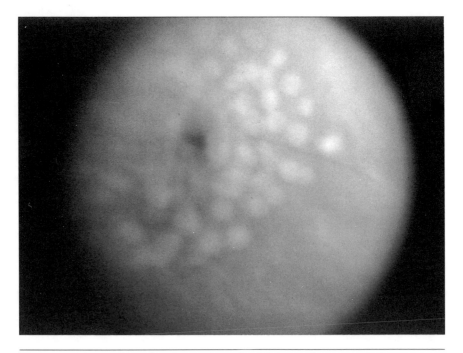

Figure 5.2 Retinal tear in a boxer treated with laser photocoagulation.

blindness may result from a sharp blow to the head (such as the impact from falling onto the canvas at the time of a knockout). Ringside physicians should realize that a boxer with cortical blindness may have no vision whatsoever, yet be totally indifferent to the visual loss and have normally reactive pupils.

Injuries to the Periorbita and Orbit

Possible boxing injuries to the periorbita and orbit include lid and soft tissue lacerations, injury to the extraocular muscles, and fractures to the orbital rim and floor.

Lid and Soft Tissue Lacerations: Lacerations to the lid and soft tissue are commonplace. Lid lacerations involving the lid margin should be repaired by an ophthalmologist or a plastic surgeon who is well versed in lid anatomy. Improper suturing of lid margin lacerations can result in scarring of the lid margin, with subsequent corneal irritation and breakdown. The physician should assume that substantial periorbital trauma is associated with intraocular injury and should consult an ophthalmologist. Damage to the levator aponeurosis may result in ptosis.

Damage to the Extraocular Muscles: Injury to these muscles may result in motility problems and diplopia. The most common muscle injured

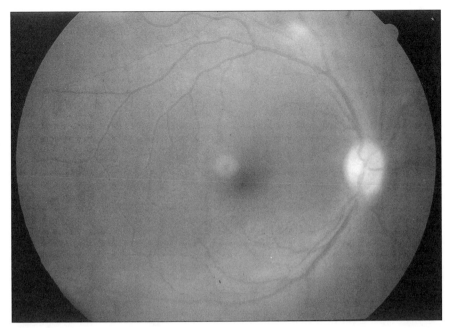

a

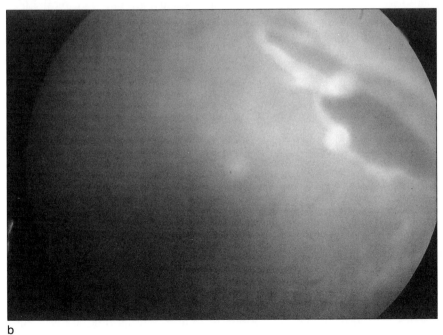

b

Figure 5.3 Retinal detachment in a boxer with 20/30 visual acuity. Only dilated fundus examination revealed the retinal pathology. Note normal-appearing posterior fundus (a) in the presence of a large peripheral retinal tear and detachment (b).

in boxers is the superior oblique, probably from damage to the trochlea. When motility disturbances are identified, the injury may have occurred to the third, fourth, or sixth cranial nerve intracranially from closed head trauma. Orbital fractures, edema, and hematoma may also restrict extraocular ocular muscle motion.

Fractures to the Orbital Rim and Orbital Floor: Such fractures do not require repair unless there is associated facial flattening, enophthalmos, or diplopia. Evaluation of the eye by an ophthalmologist is essential, as fractures of the orbit and orbital floor are commonly associated with severe and potentially blinding intraocular injury.

The Incidence of Eye Injuries in Boxing

If the usual sources are referenced, it would appear that eye injuries from boxing are extremely rare. Only 34 of a total 37,005 eye injuries resulting from sports and recreational activities in 1990 were attributed to boxing by the National Society to Prevent Blindness (1). In gathering data for the report, the National Society to Prevent Blindness used the following sources: U.S. Consumer Product Safety Commission, Directorate for Epidemiology, National Injury Information Clearinghouse, National Electronic Injury Surveillance System, and Product Summary Report—Eye Injuries Only—Calendar Year 1990.

The problem is that data and estimates supplied by these sources are based on injuries treated in hospital emergency rooms that patients say are related to products. Thus, unless a boxer with an eye injury is treated in a hospital emergency room that happens to be in the data base group of hospital emergency rooms and attributes his injury to a product (boxing glove, headgear, ring post, etc.), the injury will not be recorded and included in the annual report. Also not available from these data are the nature and severity of the injury and any long-term follow-up as to the ultimate visual result of the injury.

Another potential source would seem to be The National Eye Trauma Surveillance System (NETS), which studies perforating and penetrating eye injuries. However, as no boxing eye injuries result in penetration or actual rupture of the eye, NETS is of no value for evaluating eye injuries in boxing.

As an investigator looks through available data bases, it soon becomes apparent that there is no national or even regional comprehensive source of data regarding the incidence, severity, and long-term outcome of eye injuries from boxing. Yet it is apparent to any ophthalmologist who has examined boxers that eye injuries as a direct result of boxing are very common.

Ophthalmologists who actually care for the injured boxers realize that several factors prevent accurate counts of eye injuries due to boxing:

- Boxers tend not to be seen in hospital emergency rooms, as eye injuries are the accepted result of the sport and are usually "toughed out" with little or no treatment.
- Blinding injuries most often affect one eye, and the boxer will frequently hide the defect for fear of being disqualified from the sport.
- Other blinding eye injuries, such as glaucoma from angle recession, may occur many years after retirement from the sport and a correlation between the blindness and boxing will not be made—and if made, it will not be reported to any central monitoring agency.

Thus, if the true incidence of eye injuries to boxers is to be ascertained, one must look to smaller studies that specifically address the problem rather than large data bases that essentially ignore the sport.

Since Olympic and professional boxing are dissimilar sports, they will be considered separately.

Olympic (Amateur) Boxing

Unfortunately, very little data are available concerning eye injuries to Olympic boxers. The only study available is one conducted by Dr. David W. Sime (personal communication). In 1984, 13 Olympic boxers were given eye examinations by Dr. Sime. Of those 13, three had retinal holes or tears, probably as a result of boxing, and one had an unrelated amblyopia that reduced his best corrected vision in the amblyopic eye to 20/400. U.S. Olympic boxers have not had any regular mandated eye examination program, nor was there any follow-up on the meeting of the U.S. Olympic Committee task force on head injuries in amateur boxing held on August 20, 1983.

The instructional program at the U.S. Military Academy at West Point is fashioned after the Olympic program. Although the total injury rate for the Academy's program seems low (less than 4% injuries in 2,100 cadets who received boxing instruction between 1983 and 1985), the incidence of eye injuries is impossible to evaluate, since no asymptomatic participants had the benefit of an adequate ophthalmological examination for this study (2). Colonel John Rifile is now conducting a study at West Point to determine the incidence of ocular problems in the boxing program there.

Professional Boxing

The most reliable studies at this time involve complete eye examinations on relatively large groups of active professional boxers.

In one study 74 asymptomatic boxers in various stages of their active careers were referred to the Sports Vision Institute of Manhattan Eye, Ear & Throat Hospital on a sequential basis by the New York State Boxing Commission over a two-year period (Feb. 1984 to Feb. 1986). The boxers averaged 61 bouts with eight losses over nine years. Vision-threatening injuries (significant damage to the angle, lens, macula, or peripheral retina) occurred in 43 boxers (58%). Two boxers were actively boxing with best corrected visual acuity of 20/200 in the injured eye. Retinal tears were directly related to the total number of bouts and the number of losses. Of asymptomatic boxers, 24% had retinal tears. It was calculated by the authors that a boxer has a 20% chance of a retinal tear after five losses and a 90% chance of a retinal tear after 75 bouts (3).

A study of 284 boxers in New Jersey confirms the high incidence of eye injuries in boxing, with 19% of those dilated having retinal problems and 15% having cataracts attributable to the sport. In this series, three boxers (of whom two were world champions) had their careers ended following the need for cataract extraction (4, 5).

A study of 505 professional boxers reported at the 1991 American Academy of Ophthalmology annual meeting by Dr. Michael Goldstein confirms the high incidence of boxing-induced ocular injuries found in the studies of Giovinazzo and Smith. Dr. Goldstein has presented the largest reported series on ocular problems in boxers to date. His work shows that eye injuries are common, with the following percentages of the group studied having eye injuries: 18% retinal holes, 38.8% angle abnormalities, 5.9% posterior subcapsular cataracts.

The Prevention of Eye Injuries in Boxing

There is no question that visual loss in boxers could be substantially reduced if only the controllers and promoters of the sport would cooperate (voluntarily or otherwise) with reasonable proposals and programs to evaluate, treat, and prevent eye injuries to boxers.

The following are some possibilities for consideration and their merits and drawbacks:

• *Eliminating blows to the head*. This certainly would eliminate eye and brain injuries, but also would significantly alter the nature and appeal of the sport and has virtually no chance of acceptance by athletes, promoters, or fans.

• *Thumbless gloves*. Thumbless gloves (see Figure 5.4) or other glove designs that do not permit the thumb to extend into the "hitchhiker's position" (see Figure 5.5, page 74) would definitely help when a helmet is worn (such as in sparring). The thumb of the glove then is not able to enter the eye opening of the helmet. However, the effect of the thumbless or thumb-restrained glove on eye injuries incurred in a professional bout, in which helmets are not worn, is uncertain at this time. Only long-term, accurate data can demonstrate whether eye injuries from boxing are due to thumbing or are the result of compression and deformation of the glove face causing severe compression of the globe of the eye. High-speed photography, as has been used to analyze racquetball (6), would

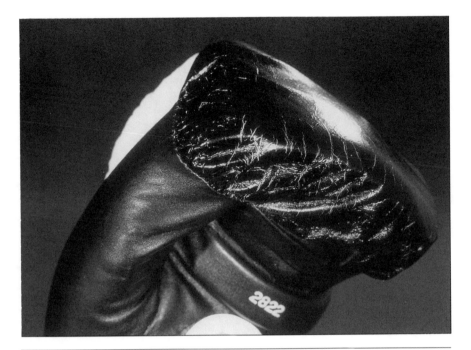

Figure 5.4   The thumbless glove.

be required to demonstrate the true deformation of various types of boxing gloves and the value of padding other than the traditional horsehair.

• *Protective helmet.* The wearing of a protective helmet and face guard (such as is worn by hockey players) during sparring sessions would effectively eliminate the risk of eye injury. However, the effect on the brain from torsional forces directed through a face guard have not been determined, and such a face guard may actually increase the chances of brain injury during sparring bouts.

• *Early detection and treatment.* While equipment changes may decrease eye injuries to boxers to some extent, the total reduction would most likely be small and delayed by many years. The main thrust toward preventing blindness and permanent disability to boxers in the near future lies in the early detection and treatment of eye injuries. Untreated injuries could lead to blindness and to prohibition from the sport of those boxers with eye conditions with a very high probability of blindness if boxing is continued.

• *American Academy of Ophthalmology recommendations.* The recommendations made in the policy statement of The American Academy of Ophthalmology should be adopted. These appear in the appendix at the end of this chapter.

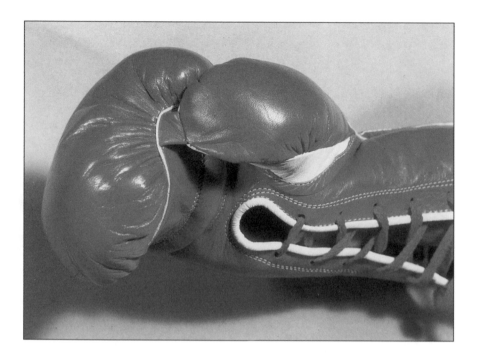

Figure 5.5 The thumb-locked glove.

Future Research and Data Collection

The incidence and prevalence of ocular injuries in boxing have been well studied in a cross-sectional study performed with prospectivity, randomization, and matched controls (3). Large anecdotal studies have confirmed these findings (4, 5). A prospective, longitudinal study is needed to follow ocular injuries in boxers over a period of years to see whether vision-threatening injuries, such as angle recession, do end in vision loss through chronic, degenerative diseases such as glaucoma.

Careful collection of data in the future may help determine whether safety measures such as the thumbless glove do reduce the incidence of vision-threatening injuries.

The disposition of the boxer after surgical repair of an ocular injury is still a matter of considerable controversy. Data on boxers who have returned to the ring after repair of a retinal detachment or removal of a cataract will greatly assist in medical judgments of these cases. The tendency of boxers to avoid follow-up care and medical scrutiny must be taken into account in any long-term prospective study.

Recent Reforms in Boxing to Prevent Ocular Injury

The American Academy of Ophthalmology has adopted a series of guidelines for reforms to prevent ocular injuries in boxing (see appendix at end of chapter). Through the Academy, ophthalmologists have begun to work on a state-by-state basis for the adoption of reforms by each state athletic commission. New York State, which has fully adopted the reforms suggested by the Academy, has led the way towards a safer boxing future and is a model for eye safety and prevention. New Jersey mandates yearly ophthalmologic examinations before granting licensure, and thumbless gloves are used in all nonchampionship fights.

Nationwide there has been no standardization of regulations, and boxers who are rejected for licensure in one state have been able to fight in other states where there is no medical requirement. Changing rules and regulations state by state is a slow and cumbersome process. A national commission or an act of Congress that would standardize requirements is desperately needed.

A high incidence of ocular injuries occurs in boxers, but many of these injuries are treatable if detected early. A complete, dilated eye examination by an ophthalmologist is necessary to diagnose ocular injuries before they can cause visual loss. Uniform regulations enacted on a nationwide level, mandating eye examinations and safety equipment, will reduce the frequency and severity of ocular injuries in boxing.

References

1. 1990 sports and recreational eye injuries. 1991 June; 2 p. Available from: National Society to Prevent Blindness, Schaumburg, IL.
2. Welch, M.J.; Sitler, M.; Kroeten, H. Boxing injuries from an instructional program. Phy. Sportsmed. 14:81-89; 1986.
3. Giovinazzo, V.J.; Yannuzzi, L.A.; Sorenson, J.A.; Delrowe, D.J.; Campbell, E.A. The ocular complications of boxing. Ophthalmology 94:587-596; 1987.
4. Smith, D.J. Ocular injuries in boxers. Paper presented at Research to prevent blindness science writers seminar in ophthalmology. New York: 1986 October.
5. Smith, D.J. Ocular injuries in boxing. In: Vinger, P.F., ed. Prevention of ocular sports injuries. International Ophthalmology Clinics. Boston: Little, Brown and Co.; 1988: p. 242-245.
6. Vinger, P.F. The eye and sports medicine. In: Duane, T.D., ed. Clinical ophthalmology. Vol. 5. Philadelphia: Harper & Row; 1985: p. 1-51.

APPENDIX

Policy Statement

REFORMS FOR THE PREVENTION OF EYE INJURIES IN BOXING*

Policy:

The American Academy of Ophthalmology recognizes the high incidence of ocular injuries in boxing and the lack of appropriate guidelines and regulations to prevent these injuries and protect participants in the sport. Severe reform measures with strict enforcement are necessary to reduce ocular injuries, promote early diagnosis and treatment, and prevent visual disability in the sport of boxing.

Background:

Serious eye injuries, such as retinal detachments, have long been known to occur in boxing.[1,2] Recent research has shown that even asymptomatic boxers, those without any visual complaints, have a high incidence of injuries that are potentially visually threatening.[3] Over half of the boxers examined had injuries that could cause a loss of vision, either acutely or insidiously.

Many of these injuries, when detected at an early stage, can be effectively treated before the onset of visual loss. This emphasizes the importance of frequent and thorough eye examinations for all boxers. In addition, examinations, including a dilated fundus examination, should be performed whenever ocular injury may have occurred.

The goal of frequent examinations is not only to diagnose and treat early injuries, but also to detect those boxers who have already suffered visual loss and to prevent any further risk to their vision by continued participation in the sport.

Guidelines:

Examination of Boxers

1. There should be specific requirements regarding ocular examinations of boxers as follows:

    a. An initial complete eye examination should be required before licensure for either amateur or professional boxing. This initial

---

*©1990 American Academy of Opthalmology, Inc. Reprinted with permission.

examination should include visual acuity, visual fields, slit-lamp biomicroscopy, intraocular pressure measurement, gonioscopy, and a dilated vitreoretinal examination including indirect ophthalmoscopy with scleral depression by an ophthalmologist.

b. A repeat, complete eye examination should be performed after one year, 6 bouts, 2 losses,[3] the stopping of a fight after an eye injury, or at the discretion of the ringside physician.

2. A mandatory, temporary suspension from sparring or boxing should be required for specific ocular pathology. When a retinal tear is identified and treated, a minimum 30-day suspension from the ring should be enforced. When a retinal detachment is treated and if a boxer is to resume his career, a minimum of 60 days mandatory suspension should be enforced. Suspensions may be individualized in consultation with the medical advisory board of each state athletic commission.

3. The minimal visual requirements for boxing should be:

a. A corrected visual acuity of 20/40 or better in each eye.
b. A full central visual field of not less than 30 degrees in each eye.

4. An ophthalmologist should serve on each state and medical boxing advisory board to advise on a boxer's eligibility for licensure.

Safety Equipment

5. There should be adopted by state and local licensing agencies adequate safety equipment to minimize ocular injuries. The thumb of most regulation boxing gloves is small enough to penetrate the orbital rim. It is an important cause of blunt ocular trauma sustained in the boxing ring. This injury can be eliminated by the use of the thumbless boxing glove. The use of the thumbless boxing glove should be mandatory not only in all amateur and professional bouts, but also in all sparring matches.

Regulations

6. There should be established in the United States a "National Registry of Boxers" for all amateur and professional boxers including sparring mates. A computer-based, central registry of this kind would be effective in recording licensed bouts and specifically noting technical knockouts, knockouts, and significant ocular injuries. When a bout is stopped because of an ocular injury, proper records and documentation should insure adequate examinations of injured boxers.

7. There should be a program of training and recertification of ringside physicians in the proper identification of serious eye injuries sustained in the ring. The diagnosis of serious eye injuries and specific criteria for suspension of a bout should be emphasized during this training period. Seminars should be planned and conducted in cooperation with

the American Association of Ringside Physicians and the American Academy of Ophthalmology.

8. There should be adopted by state and local licensing agencies a uniform code of safety requiring that a boxing match shall be stopped upon the occurrence of specified ocular symptoms or injuries such as visual field loss and blood in the anterior or posterior segment of the eye.

Summary:

A high incidence of ocular injuries occurs in boxers, but many of these injuries are treatable if detected early. A complete, dilated eye examination by an ophthalmologist is necessary to diagnose ocular injuries before they cause visual loss. Uniform regulations, enacted on a nationwide basis, mandating required eye examinations and safety equipment, will reduce the frequency and severity of ocular injuries in boxing.

Footnotes:

1. JH Doggert: "The impact of boxing on the visual apparatus," *Arch. Ophthalmol.*, 54:161-169, 1955.
2. JI Maguire and WE Benson: "Retinal injury and detachment in boxers," *J. Amer. Medical Assoc.*, 255:2451-2453, 1986.
3. VJ Giovinazzo, LA Yannuzzi, JA Sorenson, DJ Delrowe, and EA Cambell: "The ocular complications of boxing," *Ophthalmology*, 94:587-596, 1987.

Developed by: Eye Safety and Sports Ophthalmology Committee

Approved by: Board of Directors June 23, 1990

CHAPTER 6

Injuries to the Extremities, Trunk, and Head

Joseph J. Estwanik

Recently there has been a plethora of opinions on both acute and chronic brain injuries in boxing. However, little information has been available on injuries to the rest of the boxer's body. This chapter addresses this deficit by describing injury exposure and common injuries to boxers other than brain injuries.

Injury Exposure

In 1983 Demos, for the USA/Amateur Boxing Federation, conducted and completed a two-year study (1) based on the voluntary reporting system during sanctioned amateur bouts in the United States. This in-house report was based on 6,050 bouts involving 12,100 contestants. The number of injuries relayed to the authors and investigators was 174 and the calculated injury rate was 1.43%. Headgear was totally optional then and not a required safety measure. When those injuries that would have been affected by the wearing of headgear were analyzed, 22% of the traumas occurred while headgear was being worn in comparison to 78% that occurred while the protective headpiece was not being worn. Also, 53 lacerations occurred in those without headgear whereas those wearing headgear received only 20% of the total number of treated and reported lacerations.

Estwanik et al. (2) reported the total injury statistics from both the 1981 and 1982 USA/Amateur Boxing Federation Championships. This large sampling represented 547 bouts that were prospectively surveyed by the ringside physicians covering the events. Thus, 1,094 participation-risk exposures were analyzed. Table 6.1 specifically identifies the non-head injury data. The injury rate calculated from these highly competitive tournaments was 4.75%. It is historically valid to note that most of the thumb injuries seen in this study would not have occurred with the more modern thumb-attached/thumbless gloves that are now utilized in amateur boxing. Additionally, with the advent of required headgear, legislated in the mid-1980s, a tremendous decrease in the volume of facial lacerations has been evident in competitions. Formerly it was customary for a physician to bring suture kits when covering boxing events. Designated triage areas for the suturing of boxers were preplanned for most major events. Now, with the advent of headgear, it is uncommon to see lacerations of any magnitude or frequency in amateur boxing. The author has, in fact, voluntarily refrained from routinely carrying a suture kit while attending the usual tournaments unless traveling with the team on a more extended trip.

It is important to note the impact of equipment changes within one decade on these two areas of prominent exposure. With the elimination of these two "corrected" areas of trauma one could manipulate the injury statistics of Estwanik et al. to a more updated version with a 2.83% injury rate. According to some comparisons, the injury rate reported for high school football ranges as high as 46%.

Welch et al. (3) in 1986 reported on the boxing injuries sustained within an instructional program at the United States Military Academy at West Point. Boxing is an integral component of the physical development program for all male cadets and remains a required course of instruction. Throughout the two-year period covered by this report, from 1983 to 1985, about 2,100 cadets received boxing instruction, with a resulting injury rate of less than 4%. It is stated by the United States Military Program in West Point that boxing is "beneficial for the development of muscular coordination, muscular endurance, and agility. Boxing also helps cadets to react and defend themselves when physical stress is present" (3; p. 82). West Point provided accurate documentation as their program began, with an injury questionnaire, orientation discussion, notation of preexisting abnormalities, and surveillance by certified athletic trainers. When injuries did occur, a physician evaluated the cadets and completed appropriate reports. Exposure time was quite significant, with the groups totaling 23,625 hours in instructional activities and 1,680 hours in the competitive phase of the boxing program. During the instructional phase, the injury rate was 9 per 1,000 hours, while during the competitive phase the injury rate increased by a factor of five, to a total of 43 injuries per 1,000 hours of boxing. Table 6.2, page 82, summarizes the volume of injuries seen both in instructional and competitive phases of training. As expected in most sporting activities, the competitive phase poses a greater risk to the participants than the daily training. Welch et al. calculated that the injury exposure to the cadets during their competitive bouts averaged

Table 6.1 Types of Boxing Injuries at the 1981 and 1982 USA/ABF National Championships*

Injury	No.
Hand, soft tissue	**19**
Sprained thumb metacarpophalangeal collateral ligament	7
Subungual hematoma	1
Contusion and/or sprained hand	10
Sprained wrist	1
Facial lacerations	**14**
Sutured	14
Fractures	**7**
Nose	3
Ribs	1
Fifth metacarpal	2
Lunate	1
Miscellaneous	**4**
Knee effusion	1
Ankle sprain	1
Acromioclavicular joint sprain	1
Acute lumbar strain	1
Ear	**3**
Perforated lympanic membrane	2
Subperichondrial hematoma	1
Eye	**3**
Corneal abrasion	2
Subconjunctival hematoma	1
Mouth	**2**
Fractured teeth	2

*From "Amateur Boxing Injuries at the 1981 and 1982 USA/ABF National Championships" by J.J. Estwanik, M. Boitano, and N. Ari, 1984, *Physician and Sportsmedicine*, **12**(10), p. 124. Copyright 1984 by McGraw-Hill, Inc. Reprinted by permission.

3.7%, which is lower than the rates for other researched contact sports such as high school wrestling (4).

In 1990 a review of amateur boxing injuries sustained by teams training at the United States Olympic Training Center was reported by Jordan, Voy, and Stone (5). The total number of boxers could not be calculated, but the study population consisted of boxers training at the Olympic Center over a ten-year period. During this time, 447 injuries had occurred; their breakdown is listed in Table 6.3, page 83. Interestingly, cerebral injuries accounted for only 6.5% of all injuries seen, perhaps because training at the center was primarily noncompetitive aside from the usual contact made during training and sparring.

Table 6.2   Number of Days Cadets Excused From Physical Activity as a Result of Injuries Sustained During a U.S. Military Academy Boxing Program*

	Instructional phase[a]			Competitive graded bouts[b]		
	No. of injuries	Mean	Median	No. of injuries	Mean	Median
Abdomen	1	30	—	—	—	—
Ankle	5	13	11	3	16	19
Elbow	10	12	8	4	8	7
Finger	6	15	15	1	13	—
Hand	7	19	11	2	20	—
Head	18	16	15	4	15	15
Knee	3	17	14	—	—	—
Jaw	6	11	11	—	—	—
Neck	3	14	14	1	10	—
Nose	79	15	11	35	12	10
Ribs	1	7	—	—	—	—
Shoulder	56	18	14	10	20	20
Thigh	—	—	—	1	8	—
Thumb	9	18	16	4	17	10
Wrist	17	21	18	8	8	7

[a]Fifteen lessons (45 min each). [b]Four bouts (two 1-1/2 min rounds each).

*From "Boxing Injuries From an Instructional Program" by M.J. Welch, M. Sitler, and H. Kroeten, 1986, *Physician and Sportsmedicine*, **14**(9), p. 86. Copyright 1986 by McGraw-Hill, Inc. Reprinted by permission.

Enzenauer et al. (6) conducted a study evaluating boxing-related injuries in the Army over a five-year period. In a review it was calculated that 67 hospitalizations per year were attributable to boxing matches of the interunit or interservice competition variety. Those injured spent an average of five days in bed and nine days being disabled and unfit for duty. Fifty-eight percent of all the injuries were blows to the head. Some physicians have questioned the validity of the term *hospitalization* in this study as it applies to the military. It has been argued by the Amateur Boxing Federation that the criteria for hospitalization and injury observation in the military are more liberal than in the civilian sector, as discharges to family and home can be accomplished with greater ease than a soldier's return to military housing or the barracks.

Injury Analysis

With an overview of injury exposure completed, attention can now be focused towards those areas of the body that are more frequently exposed to injury during the course of training and competing.

Table 6.3   Types of Boxing Injuries at the U.S. Olympic Training Center During a 10-Year Period*

Injury site	No.	% of total injuries
Upper extremity	147	32.9
Lower extremity	107	23.9
Head and face (includes eye, ear, nose, and mouth/throat)	92	20.6
Back	31	6.9
Cerebral	29	6.5
Cervical spine, brachial plexus	23	5.1
Chest	17	3.8
Kidney	1	0.2
Total	447	100.0

*From "Amateur Boxing Injuries at the U.S. Olympic Training Center" by B.D. Jordan, R.O. Voy, and J. Stone, 1990, *Physician and Sportsmedicine*, **18**(2), p. 82. Copyright 1990 by McGraw-Hill, Inc. Reprinted by permission.

Upper Extremities

Data in Table 6.2 show that the upper extremity is at greater risk than the head (closed head injury excluded), face, lower extremities, and trunk. Analysis may be clarified if we generalize that competition places different stresses on the athlete than his training sessions. These training sessions emphasize conditioning exercises, more fully utilizing the lower extremities. During the competitions surveyed by Estwanik et al., upper extremity injuries accounted for 44% of the non-head traumas, while at the U.S. Olympic Training Center, the upper extremity was injured 33% of the time. During the instructional phase at West Point, the upper extremity was injured 48% of the time, while in their competitions, the upper extremity was injured in 46% of the mishaps. The evenness of the West Point injury rates may result from the fact that less time is spent in competition in the West Point program.

Shoulder: In the process of generating multiple, frequent, and powerful punches, the shoulder joint and its surrounding musculature create explosive accelerations. In addition, as boxers are absorbed in competition and daily training, they throw thousands upon thousands of punches, overusing the shoulder. As might be expected, rotator cuff injury, bursitis, and occasional tendinitis of the long head of the biceps can result. (Acromioclavicular and sternoclavicular injuries are not seen frequently.)

More serious shoulder injury in boxing involves subluxation or dislocation. Such an injury happens as the arm is in abduction and external rotation. This may occur as a result of a missed punch or a force applied to an arm that is awkwardly positioned or tied up by an opponent.

Elbow:　The elbow is heavily utilized in boxing, and nearly all injuries of the elbow in boxing are associated with hyperextension of that joint. The at-risk position again occurs with a missed punch as well as a misdirected blow applied to the boxer's elbow as the opponent has slid past a thrown punch. Some combination of injuries to the medial or lateral ligaments of the elbow may be present, but usually these are secondary to the main factor, which is excessive extension of the elbow. Unless the boxer falls onto the upper extremity because he slips or is knocked down, one rarely treats a fracture or dislocation.

Wrist and Hand:　Wrist injuries will certainly be seen in boxers, and the wrist is simply an important link in the chain of events as the upper arm delivers a blow. The wrist has been customarily supported by the use of wraps prior to punches being thrown. Most boxers will require their wrists to be supportively wrapped in a gauze or linen strap. Temporary cloth straps are routinely used for training purposes and can be applied rather rapidly. However, prior to a competition, an experienced boxer will insist on having a qualified coach or trainer precisely apply a combination of gauze and tape. The soft surgical gauze utilized is generally two inches wide and ranges from 10 to 12 yards in length. A skilled coach wrapping the hands and wrists is akin to the athletic trainer masterfully weaving tape about an ankle. The padding over the knuckles must be correct but must not limit the ability to flex all joints of the hand into the proper punching position. Of course, the tape also crosses the wrist to protectively reinforce this joint. A final cloth adhesive tape is then applied over the wrap to seal it in place and further strengthen it.

Prior to competitions, boxing officials examine each hand wrap to see that it is properly applied and scroll their initials on the tape to certify this inspection. The boxer can place no adhesive tape over the knuckles. The hand wrap is meant only to protect the boxer's hand, not to emphasize the force of the blow. The inspection ensures that the gauze has not been moistened and that no unauthorized substances are present in the wrap.

Despite the protection of the glove and wrap, compression or flexion extension injuries will occur. Usually these are sprains of the wrist, but as a rule, the author distrusts the term *sprained wrist* and is overly cautious in ruling out an occult fracture of the carpals or insidious rotatory instabilities. Fractures of the metacarpal are much easier to diagnose, with localized swelling and point tenderness. An x-ray is usually sufficient to document these fractures. Injuries to the metacarpophalangeal (MCP) joints of the boxer's hand are very common and simply result from the force of the blow onto the punching portion of the hand. With the forces properly applied, the majority of the impact should be delivered to the more stable second and third metacarpal heads, while misdirected punches land towards the fifth metacarpal unit. Certainly a fracture inhibits a boxer's ability to punch until adequate healing has occurred.

Directly related to the force applied during the punching mechanism, synovitis and extensor tendon subluxations are more frequent complications in boxing than in other athletic endeavors. The author has actually witnessed a punch thrown so hard that the involved boxer acutely dislocated the extensor tendon from its central position over the third metacarpal head. The boxer ineffectively continued boxing the third round and finished the competition. Upon unwrapping the hand, he was unable to straighten this finger, as the extensor tendon was lying in the gutter between metacarpal heads. This was temporarily and manually reduced, but it eventually required surgical centralization and repair that later allowed the athlete to win a medal in the Olympic games. An accumulation of hard punches will also cause synovitis of the MCP joints, which responds to rest, icing, anti-inflammatories, and gentle physical therapy.

Posner and Ambrose, in an article, "Boxer's Knuckle: Dorsal Capsular Rupture of the Metacarpophalangeal Joint of a Finger" (7), described their experience with this injury in six patients. Dorsal capsular rupture damages the sagittal fibers of the extensor tendon mechanism, with further trauma resulting in the rupture of the underlying joint capsule. It is clinically important to differentiate the deeper capsular rupture from the less severe dorsal hood injury, as the latter may respond to conservative treatment while the former requires a surgical repair.

The thumb was classically a weak point for the boxer prior to the creation of the thumbless or thumb-attached glove. As a blow was blocked or the boxer missed a punch, the thumb unit was caught and forced into excessive abduction. Ligamentous tear, synovitis, or fracture resulted. Luckily this injury is one that has been recognized, documented, understood, and successfully prevented. The simple redesign of equipment has quite dramatically improved this situation.

Lower Extremities

Few lower extremity injuries occur in boxers during their performance, aside from an ankle sprain that complicates an uncontrolled fall or slip. It is extremely unlikely that a boxer will fall out of the ring, but the boxer's foot can slide beyond the ropes and extend past the padded surface of the mat above the official's tables.

Many lower extremity injuries can be prevented by proper supervision and attention to detail when setting up the ring. The ropes must be of the proper height and tension and must allow the apron of the ring floor to extend not less than two feet beyond the ropes. The canvas mat should also be evaluated by boxing personnel for proper tension to prevent ankle- and knee-twisting injuries. A very occasional meniscus or ligamental injury to the knee may occur with improper torque applied to that extremity.

While upper extremities have a greater tendency to be injured from the acute trauma of competition, the lower extremities will often suffer wear and tear from training methods that cause chronic overuse. Stress fractures and patellar chondromalacia can be prevented by proper supervision of the aerobic and the running portions of the training program. Boxers should wear appropriately designed running shoes when conditioning, then switch back to the usual boxing footwear when exercising the fundamentals of boxing. Running shoes were made for running and boxing shoes were made for boxing!

Trunk

Some low-back injuries will be precipitated by the multiple repetitions of abdominal exercising and the trunk twisting that is necessary for generating the punch. Avoiding harsh training techniques may prevent some chronic lumbar injuries; the remainder of injuries to the lumbar spine are fairly accidental.

The cervical spine is obviously subject to direct stresses from blows delivered to the head or falls if the boxer is knocked unconscious. Thus, the boxer must develop his neck musculature to the fullest extent to protect the spine. Strong hypertrophied neck muscles act as a check-rein against the acceleration forces known to cause concussion. Strengthening of the neck musculature must be done properly, stressing reasonable ranges of motion and isometric techniques. Improper compressive forces and heavy weights will likely cause eventual disc degeneration in the cervical spine. Boitano (8) described an unusual ligamentous injury of the upper cervical spine that was incurred by a boxer during the 1984 Los Angeles Olympics. This boxer had been struck in the back of the head by an illegal blow, which was noted by doctors and officials while reviewing tapes of the match.

Rib fractures, rib contusions, and costochondral injuries tremendously hamper the boxer's ability to train and compete. However, training should focus on strong abdominal and spine musculature. Appropriate training methods and carefully supervised sparring and competitions should protect the spine from chronic and acute injury.

Head and Face

When we consider ear injuries of the boxer, most now are tympanic membrane ruptures. Even with the headgear in place, a punch improperly thrown with the palmar portion of the glove (a "slap") or a full-fisted blow to the ear can create a vacuum and rupture the eardrum. Analgesics, oral antibiotics, and a protective cotton plug should allow proper healing. It is important to avoid splashing any water into the ear canal. The healing may need to be checked by an ENT specialist, although usually the eardrum will re-epithelialize under the proper conditions. No boxing, only fitness training, is allowed until the healing process is completed.

Cauliflower ear deformity has become less prevalent with the protection of headgear. Rapid drainage and packing or suturing of hematomas in the ear will prevent the deposition of scar cartilage that is the basis of the deformity.

As long as blows have been thrown, the nose has somehow always been in the way. Isn't the old-time boxer characterized by the flattened but proudly worn nose? In most cases, epistaxis (simple nasal bleeding) is the only resulting trauma, but in the past few years, physicians have checked more closely for septal hematoma and septal deviations. The nasal complex, including the septal structures, must be thoroughly inspected following an injury. Boxers who have frustrating episodes of frequent but benign epistaxis can be evaluated by an ENT surgeon who can, if necessary, cauterize the superficial plexus of veins.

References

1. Demos, M. *Mouthpiece*, 2(3):20; 1983.
2. Estwanik, J.J.; Boitano, M.; Ari, N. Amateur boxing injuries at the 1981 and 1982 USA/ABF National Championships. Phy. Sportsmed. 12:123-128; 1984.
3. Welch M.J.; Sitler, M.; Kroeten, H. Boxing injuries from an instructional program. Phy. Sportsmed. 14:81-90; 1986.
4. Estwanik, J.J.; Rovere, G.D. Wrestling injuries in North Carolina high schools. Phy. Sportsmed. 11:100-108; 1986.
5. Jordan, B.D.; Voy, R.O.; Stone, J. Amateur boxing injuries at the U.S. Olympic Training Center. Phy. Sportsmed. 18:80-90; 1990.
6. Enzenauer, R.W.; Montrey, J.S.; Enzenauer, R.J.; Mauldin, W.M. Boxing-related injuries in the U.S. Army, 1980 through 1985. JAMA 261:1463-1466; 1989.
7. Posner, M.A.; Ambrose, L. Boxer's knuckle: Dorsal capsular rupture of the metacarpophalangeal joint of a finger. Joint Hand Surg. 14A:229-236; 1989.
8. Boitano, M. Cervical spine in boxing unusual ligamentous injury in olympic boxer and review of the literature. Hungar. Rev. Sports Med. 27(3):175-180; 1986.

CHAPTER 7

The Ringside Physician's Role*

Joseph J. Estwanik
Francis G. O'Connor

Boxing is a sport that has long been criticized by physicians because of its potential to cause serious injury (1-10). The sport of amateur boxing, however, has been unparalleled in the quest to maintain the safety of its competitors. Amateur boxing organizations have been instrumental in implementing rule and equipment changes that have served to promote the welfare of the athlete (11, 12). In addition, boxing mandates physician attendance at all competitions, with the medical doctor having the authority to stop a bout at any time. This chapter will detail the role of the amateur boxing team physician and provide the health care professional with guidelines and information necessary to care for the boxing athlete.

The physician's role in boxing can be divided into two phases: 1) the preparticipation examination and 2) ringside physician duties. The ringside physician's duties can be further subdivided into the pre-bout examination, ringside responsibilities, and post-bout evaluation. Additional duties may be assumed by the traveling team physician when the team leaves the U.S.

---

*This chapter was taken in part from "Boxing: The Preparticipation Evaluation" by F.G. O'Connor and J.B. Tucker, 1991, *Military Medicine*, **156**, pp. 391-395. Copyright 1991 by the Association of Military Surgeons of the United States. Adapted by permission.

Preparticipation Exam

The preparticipation exam should ideally be performed four to six weeks prior to the onset of athletic participation. This time period allows sufficient opportunity for the athlete to correct specific conditions detected during the preparticipation examination that may require further evaluation or treatment. A recently completed standard physical examination does not suffice for preparticipation clearance because of the unique aspects of the boxing evaluation.

The history and physical examination should be performed in a private, quiet, well-lighted room, with the athlete in shorts. The examination should be individualized, as opposed to en masse screening. En masse screening has not been shown to reduce the incidence of injuries or prevent sudden death (13, 14).

Medical/Surgical History

As with nearly all examinations, the history is perhaps the most critical element. The past medical/surgical history should be designed to quickly ascertain major aspects of an individual's health history. As evidenced by the list of disqualifying conditions (Figure 7.1), some prior surgical procedures, as well as chronic medical conditions, may be contraindications to participation. The family history may alert one to investigate for a specific inheritable condition that may predispose the individual to injury. Examples include a family history of asymmetric septal hypertrophy, sudden cardiac death in a primary relative, osteogenesis imperfecta, Marfan's syndrome, neurofibromatosis, and bleeding disorders. Clues obtained through the family history will additionally help direct the physical examination and laboratory assessment. The remainder of the history is a guided review of systems that is designed to detect specific disqualifying conditions, as well as conditions that may warrant further evaluation. While all aspects of the evaluation will be discussed, particular emphasis will be placed on the central nervous system and cardiovascular assessments, as these represent areas of greatest potential risk.

Vital Signs

Vital signs represent the only aspect of the examination that may be performed by a trained nonphysician. Vital signs should include visual acuity, height, weight, and blood pressure. Blood pressure should be appropriate for age. For children under 10 years of age, 130/75 is the upper limit of normal, while for youngsters 10 to 15, the limit is 140/80 mmHg (13). In adults, USA Boxing mandates that blood pressure greater than or equal to 150/100 requires disqualification. Hypertension of any nature requires further evaluation before participation can be allowed.

General

Acute infection (respiratory, genitourinary, infectious mononucleosis, hepatitis, active rheumatic fever, active tuberculosis)

Obvious physical immaturity in comparison with other competitors in the same group

Hemorrhagic disease (hemophilia, purpura, other serious bleeding disorders)

Anemia (severe)—address etiology, such as gastrointestinal bleeding, sickle cell trait, or thalassemia

Diabetes mellitus—poor control

Malignancy—individualize by diagnosis and phase

Hyperthyroidism (not controlled)

HEENT

Documented history of retinal detachment

Uncorrected vision of > 20/60 in one or both eyes or > 20/400 in at least one eye

Blindness of one eye

Congenital glaucoma

Previous radical mastoid surgery

Severe hearing loss—no consensus, so up to individual physician

Skin

Boils, impetigo, herpes simplex, pediculosis

Respiratory system

Tuberculosis (active or symptomatic)

Asthma (poor control)

Recurrent pneumothorax without pleurodiesis

Hemoptysis

Pulmonary insufficiency—individualize

Cardiovascular system

Organic hypertension

Uncontrolled hypertension $\geq$ 150/100

Asymmetric septal hypertrophy (IHSS)

Third-degree heart block

(continued)

Figure 7.1 Boxing disqualifying conditions.[12,15-17]
From "Boxing: The Preparticipation Evaluation" by F.G. O'Connor and J.B. Tucker, 1991, *Military Medicine*, **156**, p. 392. Copyright 1991 by the Association of Military Surgeons of the United States. Reprinted by permission.

Figure 7.1 *(continued)*

Cardiovascular system *(continued)*

Valvular or cyanotic heart disease

Coarctation of aorta

Recent carditis

Persistent patent ductus arteriosus

History of cardiac surgery

Significant arrhythmia

Thromboembolic disease

Mitral valve prolapse—individualize

Abdomen

Hepatomegaly, splenomegaly

Jaundice

Hepatitis

Mononucleosis—active

Palpable tenderness/masses

Active ulcer disease, rectal bleeding

Inguinal or incisional hernia

Genitourinary

Absence of one kidney

Undescended or atrophic testicle

Inguinal or femoral hernia/hydrocele

Acute nephritis/nephrotic syndrome

Chronic renal disease

Musculoskeletal system

Symptomatic abnormalities or inflammation

Spondylolisthesis/spondylosis with pain

Inflammatory diseases (collagen-vascular)

Rheumatoid arthritis, ankylosing spondylitis

Swollen joints, fractures, recurrent dislocations

Primary muscular dystrophy

(continued)

Figure 7.1 *(continued)*

Central nervous system

History of previous serious head trauma or repeated concussions

Brain-meningeal scarring (subdural or epidural bleeds, depressed fracture, hydrocephalus, Berry aneurysm, previous craniotomy)

Seizure disorder

Posttraumatic seizure disorders

A-V malformation

Degenerative or demyelinating disorders

Well-controlled essential hypertension is not a contraindication to contact sports activity (14).

Head, Eye, Ear, Nose, Throat

USA Boxing requires that all boxers have adequate vision. A boxer with corrected visual acuity of worse than 20/60 in either eye, regardless of its cause, shall be disqualified. USA Boxing recommends that all boxers have a complete ophthalmologic evaluation at least yearly, as retinal tears, minor detachments, and glaucoma can exist undetected (11, 12). A complete ophthalmologic evaluation, however, is not required for preparticipation clearance. In addition to congential glaucoma and a history of retinal detachment, blindness in one eye or significantly decreased acuity in one eye (greater than 20/400) requires disqualification.

Anisocoria, which is present in approximately one of four persons, needs to be noted (18). The etiology of acquired anisocoria requires investigation prior to permitting participation. Congential anisocoria is not a contraindication to boxing.

The tympanic membranes must be examined to ensure that they are intact. The ability to hear commands is critical to the evaluation of the impaired boxer, so the precompetition state needs to be accurately documented. The presence of the occasional cauliflower ear, be it acute or chronic, should be noted, as protective headgear must fit securely and comfortably. Deaf and mute boxers who can pass a physical exam are eligible to compete.

The nares should be examined for the presence of hematomas and a deviated or perforated septum. While deviation is not a contraindication to boxing, functional impairment should be noted and individualized.

Face/Mouth

The physician should examine the mouth for loose teeth and tender areas; broken teeth and severe caries require referral to a dentist. While not a

USA Boxing consideration for disqualification, broken and loose teeth should receive dental attention before participation is permitted. The presence of a dental prosthesis needs to be noted and participation individualized. Previous radical mastoid surgery requires disqualification (14). Young boxers who have parental permission and a dentist-molded mouthpiece are authorized to compete wearing braces.

Pulmonary

The chest should be examined for any deformities, pulsations, or retractions. Pectus excavatum should be noted, but is not a contraindication to contact activity. Controlled asthma is not a contraindication to boxing. The International Olympic Committee has had difficulty in its approach to medication used in the treatment of asthma; B-agonists are of concern because they are considered stimulants. Currently, the use of the following B-2-agonists is permitted in the aerosol form only: terbutaline, albuterol, metaproterenol, and tornalate. Drugs such as cromolyn sodium, aminophylline, theophylline, beclamethasone, and atropine sulfate are safe to use. Corticosteriods are permitted. Use, dose, and route of administration of corticosteroids, however, must be documented and justified by the athlete's physician (12).

Abdominal

The physician should examine for organomegaly and areas of tenderness. Specific disqualifying conditions include a single testicle, single kidney, or the presence of a large or symptomatic inguinal or incisional hernia. Splenomegaly is a contraindication to contact sports activity, and it must be ruled out where there exists a history of infectious mononucleosis. The Tanner stage should be noted, as obvious physical immaturity in comparison to other competitors mandates disqualification (13). The examination should also include inspection for previous scars and surgeries. It is not necessary to perform a rectal examination for athletes under age 40 unless there is a history of rectal bleeding (14). However, the anal area may be inspected for external hemorrhoids and fissures. Jaundice should be noted and further work-up initiated prior to permitting participation.

Cardiovascular

The physician needs to perform the cardiovascular examination carefully and thoroughly. The purpose of the examination is to identify conditions that may pose an absolute or relative contraindication to boxing participation. The physician must combine a thorough review of the past medical history and cardiovascular review of systems with a comprehensive physical examination to rule out those conditions that may predispose the athlete to sudden cardiac death.

The frequency of sudden cardiac death in athletes is extremely low (19). The causes of sudden death in athletes are generally age related. Maron's landmark work evaluated sudden death in young competitive athletes (less than 35 years of age) and older athletes (35 years of age and older). Maron found that over half of the sudden death cases in young athletes are secondary to hypertrophic cardiomyopathy. Other causes in this age group include congenital coronary artery anomalies, ruptured aorta, idiopathic left ventricular hypertrophy, and myocarditis. Sudden death in older athletes is usually due to coronary artery disease, rarely resulting from congenital heart disease (20).

The past medical history should be focused on previous work-up and diagnosis. Absolute contraindications to boxing include the following: a history of cardiac surgery, third-degree heart block, hemodynamically significant valvular heart disease, coarcation of the aorta, persistent patent ductus arteriosus, and significant coronary artery disease (12, 13, 16, 17). This list is not all-inclusive, and individual cases should be discussed with a cardiologist or sports medicine specialist.

Relative contraindications include the mitral valve prolapse syndrome and significant arrhythmias. Mitral valve prolapse requires individualization. Athletes with mitral valve prolapse and a history of exertional syncope, exertional chest pain, or sudden cardiac death in a primary relative should be prohibited from boxing, pending comprehensive cardiac evaluation. In addition, mitral valve prolapse associated with dilitation of the ascending aorta, prolonged Q-T interval, significant mitral regurgitation, or significant ventricular arrhythmias also requires investigation to determine whether or not participation may be permitted (21). Further evaluation might include stress testing to evaluate the athlete's rhythm response to exercise in order to ensure that there is not hemodynamic compromise (13). Paroxysmal supraventricular tachyarrhythmias, including the Wolf-Parkinson-White syndrome, should not prevent an athlete from participation. Again, however, an exercise stress test should be considered, and the case should be discussed with a cardiologist or sports medicine specialist.

The review of systems allows the physician to identify those athletes who may be predisposed to sudden cardiac death. The physician should inquire into the following areas: syncope or presyncope, fatigue, dizziness, chest pain, dyspnea, palpitations, and a history of sudden cardiac death in a primary relative. Syncope can be characteristic of both aberrant left coronary artery and asymmetric septal hypertrophy (IHSS). Positive responses to questions about any of these should raise the physician's suspicion of possible underlying heart disease. Family history of a sudden death should alert the examiner to asymmetric septal hypertrophy. Physical examination and diagnostic testing, to include echocardiogram, ECG, chest x-rays, and stress testing, can then be utilized to determine if further evaluation by a cardiologist is necessary.

The physical examination must be performed in a quiet setting so that subtle abnormalities may be discovered. The physician must carefully identify S_1 and S_2 and then note the presence of accompanying gallops, rhythm disturbances, murmurs, snaps, and clicks. A systolic heart murmur is present on auscultation in 30 to 50% of athletes (19). The physician who is responsible for auscultation of the athlete must determine whether the murmur is functional or organic. The most common functional murmur appearing in athletes under age 25 is the Still's murmur (19). The Still's murmur is a high-pitched, early-peaking, midsystolic murmur with a vibratory quality that is heard best along the lower left sternal border. Its etiology is undetermined. The intensity of the murmur decreases with standing or valsalva. This is in direct contrast to the murmur of IHSS. Maneuvers that decrease left ventricular volume, such as standing, valsalva, and exercise, increase obstruction and enhance the murmur of IHSS. Maneuvers that increase left ventricular volume, such as squatting, soften the murmur (13). Other abnormalities that require further investigation include holosystolic murmurs, all diastolic murmurs, fixed S_2 splitting, and differences in arm/leg pulses and pressure (the last suggesting coarctation of the aorta). Experience is the best guide to distinguishing benign from potentially serious murmurs; however, echocardiogram, CXR, and ECG are helpful. The reader is referred to other sources for more detailed discussion on the interpretation of cardiac auscultation in the athlete (13, 14, 19). Additionally, an invaluable guide to the physician performing preparticipation examinations is a reprint of the 16th Bethesda Conference Regarding Cardiovascular Abnormalities and Eligibility for Competition (21).

Skin

The physician needs to examine the entire integument. Boils, impetigo, active herpetic lesions, and pediculosis are all absolute contraindications to boxing. Pustular acne is a relative contraindication to contact and needs to be individualized. Pallor suggesting anemia mandates laboratory assessment.

Musculoskeletal

The examiner should note body symmetry, as well as generalized strength, flexibility, and range of motion. Particular emphasis should be placed on the cervical spine. Because of the difficulty in determining playability following a cervical injury, it is recommended that a neck profile (assessment of cervical strength and range of motion) be completed during the preparticipation evaluation (14). Neck pain, crepitus, or decreased range of motion suggests the need for an x-ray. Evidence of joint laxity, instability, or the induction of radicular symptoms with range of motion testing warrants further evaluation prior to permitting participation.

Prior orthopedic injury/surgery is not an absolute contraindication to boxing. Each injury should be individualized and assessed for functional impairment. It should always be appreciated that a history of previous injury appears to be a risk factor for subsequent injury. Even the slightest remark about a prior minor injury should prompt the examiner to perform a careful assessment.

The hands, elbows, and shoulders are commonly the focus of boxing injury. A missed jab during a boxing match can lead to a chip of the olecranon ("boxer's elbow") or an anterior shoulder dislocation. Accordingly, the examiner should note anterior shoulder laxity/apprehension, as well as elbow tenderness and range of motion. A "boxer's fracture" is a fracture of the fifth metacarpal neck, usually occurring as a result of a punching injury. (The name is a misnomer; an unskilled fighter is more likely to experience such a fracture.) The physician should examine the hands closely for swelling and tenderness of the MCP joints and extensor tendon malposition associated with chronic capsulitis from punching. The upper extremity is also subject to overuse injuries (including the effects of strength training). The examiner should be thorough in evaluating for rotator cuff tendinitis and elbow contractures.

The preparticipation examination should also note stigmata that might suggest use of anabolic steroids. Side effects of steroid use include facial and body acne, testicular atrophy, breast enlargement, and premature baldness. Anabolic steroids are prohibited by the International Olympic Committee, and suspicion of their use warrants further evaluation (12).

Neurologic

The neurologic evaluation must incorporate a thorough past medical history, a thoughtful review of central nervous system symptoms, and a comprehensive neurologic examination. The history may often signal neurologic compromise and vulnerability before subtle signs are appreciated by even the most skillful clinician.

An initial minimum compendium of questions would explore the following areas: Is there a history of seizures? If so, what is the etiology and how well are the convulsions controlled? Is there a history of any neurosurgery or conditions that might imply brain or meningeal scarring? Is there a history of concussion? The review of systems must include history of new, changing, or debilitating headaches; awkwardness or disequilibrium; irritability, confusion, memory lapses, or personality changes; nausea or anorexia; paresthesias; diplopia or other visual symptoms; and malaise.

There are no data to suggest that those with pharmacologically well-controlled (no seizure in more than 12 months) idiopathic seizures must be restricted from contact sports (22-24). However, there is consensus that posttraumatic convulsions, particularly those following penetrating trauma, are an absolute contraindication to any further contact sport competition, including boxing (17, 25). Similarly, most authors believe that a past history of a third-degree concussion or multiple second-degree concussions (17, 25-27), previous neurosurgery, aneurysm, A-V malformation, depressed skull fracture, or subdural or epidural hematoma precludes further contact endeavors (17, 25-27).

A positive review of systems revealing symptoms in any of the areas described, even in the face of a normal neurologic examination, requires further evaluation to include computerized tomography or magnetic resonance imaging, or both, and electroencephalography before further training or competition is permitted.

The neurologic examination must be thorough and should include examination of mental status; careful visualization of the optic fundus; pupillary exam and careful documentation of pupillary asymmetry (anisocoria) as a congenital condition versus a sign of increased intracranial pressure; cranial nerve evaluation with particular attention to the extraocular muscles; and thorough evaluations of gait, sensory, and cerebellar function. Even subtle abnormalities in the neurologic examination require restriction from contact until further evaluation can be completed.

Laboratory Evaluation

In addition to the history and physical examination, laboratory tests may be indicated. Most practitioners would agree that routine lab tests in an asymptomatic population are not warranted (12, 13, 16, 17). This posture is supported by USA Boxing (12). Any diagnostic studies should be ordered only as indicated.

Disqualification

Figure 7.1 lists those conditions that commonly support disqualification. This list, constructed principally from *The Physician's Ringside Manual* and current sports medicine literature, is not all-inclusive (12). The list is intended to provide guidelines to the examining physician, not a rigid summation. The ultimate decision for participation lies with the examining physician. When in doubt, the certifying physician can consult with an appropriate specialist or contact a physician with a particular expertise in boxing.

Documentation

Documentation of the preparticipation physical examination is of immense importance. The medical record not only fulfills legal requirements, but also serves as a valuable reference for future evaluation of the athlete. There currently does not exist a uniform process of documenting the preparticipation evaluation in boxing. Lombardo et al. have recently designed a preparticipation evaluation form that has been endorsed by the American Academies of Family Practice and Pediatrics (Figure 7.2) (28). It is our opinion that this form should be considered for endorsement by USA Boxing. The safety of amateur boxers can only be enhanced by standardization of the preparticipation examination process.

Ringside Physician's Duties

The ringside physician's duties can sequentially be divided into four categories: pre-bout planning, pre-bout examination, ringside responsibilities, and post-bout evaluation. To simplify the process, USA Boxing publishes not only an *Official Rules Book* (biannually), but also a *Ringside Physician's Certification Manual* that details and specifies, in quite generous detail, the obligations of the ringside physician. We would list familiarization with these two publications as a responsibility of a ringside physician.

Pre-Bout Planning

Before walking onto the premises, the doctor should have previously discussed with the organizers and officials of the bout the contingencies for the evacuation of emergency cases. Most important is the availability, if not the on-site presence, of an ambulance or EMT unit. Usually the organizers of the event can work out financial arrangements with the local rescue squad or fire department or can barter admission tickets so an emergency vehicle is stationed at the bout. The EMT personnel are treated as important members of the event and are given choice seating arrangements, preferably at ringside. An evacuation route from ringside through the arena to the ambulance, and from there to the appropriate emergency room, should be determined before the event.

The physician needs to identify the nearest emergency rooms or hospitals, have their phone numbers handy, know where the phones are located, and have priority for use of the phones. He or she should inform the emergency room or hospital staff if a boxer needs to be transferred to them.

Even though the tournament or bout organizers are more familiar with the mechanical construction of the ring, it is also the physician's duty to check the ring for appropriate stability, rope tension, and adequate ring apron size. A 16- to 20-foot-square ring should be present with a 24-inch apron and adequately padded posts. No dangerous seams or defects in the canvas mat should be present to cause the boxer to trip or fall. The mat should be sanitary and free of obvious dust and grit. The ring floor should be a wooden base covered by 1 inch of foam or ensolite padding. There must be four covered ring ropes under appropriate tension. At least two spacer ties that run vertically between the ropes should be placed on each side of the ring to prevent a boxer's falling through the

Preparticipation Physical Evaluation

History

Name _____ Sex _____ Age _____ Date _____

Grade _____ Sport _____ Date of birth _____

Personal physician _____

Address _____ Physician's phone _____

Explain "Yes" answers below:

	Yes	No
1. Have you ever been hospitalized?	☐	☐
Have you ever had surgery?	☐	☐
2. Are you presently taking any medications or pills?	☐	☐
3. Do you have any allergies (medicine, bees or other stinging insects)?	☐	☐
4. Have you ever passed out during or after exercise?	☐	☐
Have you ever been dizzy during or after exercise?	☐	☐
Have you ever had chest pain during or after exercise?	☐	☐
Do you tire more quickly than your friends during exercise?	☐	☐
Have you ever had high blood pressure?	☐	☐
Have you ever been told that you have a heart murmur?	☐	☐
Have you ever had racing of your heart or skipped heartbeats?	☐	☐
Has anyone in your family died of heart problems or a sudden death before age 50?	☐	☐
5. Do you have any skin problems (itching, rashes, acne)?	☐	☐
6. Have you ever had a head injury?	☐	☐
Have you ever been knocked out or unconscious?	☐	☐
Have you ever had a seizure?	☐	☐
Have you ever had a stinger, burner, or pinched nerve?	☐	☐
7. Have you ever had heat or muscle cramps?	☐	☐
Have you ever been dizzy or passed out in the heat?	☐	☐
8. Do you have trouble breathing or do you cough during or after activity?	☐	☐
9. Do you use any special equipment (pads, braces, neck rolls, mouth guard, eye guards, etc.)?	☐	☐

10. Have you had any problems with your eyes or vision? .... ☐ ☐

    Do you wear glasses or contacts or protective eye wear? .... ☐ ☐

11. Have you ever sprained, strained, dislocated, fractured, or broken or had repeated swelling or other injuries of any
    bones or joints? .... ☐ ☐

    ☐ Head   ☐ Shoulder   ☐ Thigh   ☐ Neck   ☐ Elbow   ☐ Knee   ☐ Chest

    ☐ Forearm   ☐ Shin/calf   ☐ Back   ☐ Wrist   ☐ Ankle   ☐ Hip   ☐ Hand   ☐ Foot

12. Have you had any other medical problems (infectious mononucleosis, diabetes, etc.)? .... ☐ ☐

13. Have you had a medical problem or injury since your last evaluation? .... ☐ ☐

14. When was your last tetanus shot? _____

    When was your last measles immunization? _____

15. When was your first menstrual period? _____

    When was your last menstrual period? _____

    What was the longest time between your periods last year? _____

Explain "Yes" answers: _____

_____

I hereby state that, to the best of my knowledge, my answers to the above questions are correct.

Date _____

Signature of athlete _____

Signature of parent/guardian _____

(continued)

Figure 7.2   Preparticipation physical evaluation.

From Preparticipation Physical Evaluation (monograph). Kansas City, MO: American Academy of Family Physicians, American Academy of Pediatrics, American Medical Society for Sports Medicine, American Orthopaedic Society for Sports Medicine, American Osteopathic Academy of Sports Medicine, 1992.

Figure 7.2 *(continued)*

Physical Examination

Name _____

Height _____   Weight _____   BP _____   Age _____   Date _____

Vision R 20/ _____   L 20/ _____   Corrected: Y / N   Pulse _____   Pupils _____   Date of birth _____

		Normal	Abnormal findings	Initials
Limited	Cardiopulmonary			
	Pulses			
	Heart			
	Lungs			
	Tanner stage	1	2 3 4 5	
	Skin			
Complete	Abdominal			
	Genitalia			
	Musculoskeletal			
	Neck			
	Shoulder			
	Elbow			
	Wrist			
	Hand			
	Back			

Knee		
Ankle		
Foot		
Other		

Clearance:

A. Cleared

B. Cleared after completing evaluation/rehabilitation for: _____

C. Not cleared for: ❑ Collision

❑ Contact

❑ Noncontact _____ Strenuous _____ Moderately strenuous _____ Nonstrenuous

Due to: _____

Recommendation: _____

_____

_____

_____

Name of physician _____ Date _____

Address _____ Phone _____

Signature of physician _____

ropes. The senior author has actually been present at a major tournament during which one of the rings collapsed. Fortunately, no injuries resulted. A diagram for ring setup is included (see Figure 7.3).

After introducing himself to the officials, the timekeeper, the emergency personnel, and the referees, the physician should sit directly at ringside. He should be close to one of the neutral corners, with an unobstructed view away from the corner post padding. Steps should be present at this corner for rapid and easy access into the ring, not only for emergencies, but also for the more frequent minor evaluations. Oxygen and a spine board should be hidden underneath the ring for easy access without visibility.

It also is useful to designate a somewhat remote observation area near the locker room. This area can be used for completing more detailed evaluation of a boxer away from the pressures and noise of the crowd.

Pre-Bout Examination

A basic guideline by USA Boxing legislates a mandatory pre-bout physician examination on the day of the competition. It is most appropriate to

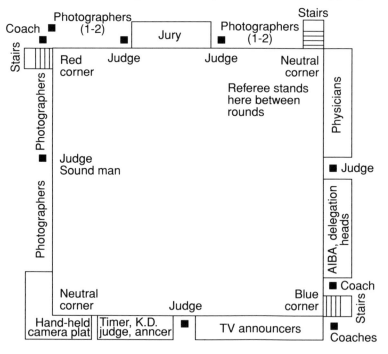

A table big enough for at least two (three is ideal) physicians is placed adjacent to one of the neutral corners. In addition, a set of steps must be placed next to the table to enable the physician to quickly mount the apron without obstruction.

Figure 7.3 Diagram for ring setup for ringside physician.
From *USA/ABF Safety Awareness Manual* (p. 53) by USA/ABF, 1988, Colorado Springs: USA/ABF. Copyright 1988 by USA/ABF. Adapted by permission.

coordinate this exam with the officials so that it occurs during weigh-ins. Sometimes it may be convenient to direct the boxers to the physician's office. However, most circumstances produce examinations at the arena during weigh-ins immediately prior to the competition. The object of this evaluation is to ensure that the competitor is healthy and to circumvent any problem during the actual competition.

At this point, the authors might propose a lofty goal and suggest that a totally comprehensive evaluation of all boxers be compulsively accomplished. However, in a practical sense, a pertinent evaluation can be accomplished in just a few minutes. A series of neurologic questions to ascertain any preexisting subdural hematoma, recent history of fever or illness, or use of medication (drug usage) is important. One should also evaluate the nutrition/hydration status of the boxer, since "making weight" is an integral component of the boxing game. The ringside physician should eventually begin to feel comfortable enough in performing these physicals that he eases into rapport with each boxer. The physician should communicate to the boxer that he is there to assist and protect the boxer, not to stop the bout. Some boxers will come to the preexamination not psychologically prepared to box and looking for a way out. By opening communication with each boxer, the physician can recognize such situations and give boxers a face-saving, comfortable, medical reason not to compete that night.

Casual remarks, hints, and questions by the ringside physician will diminish some of the boxer's anxiety and let the physician evaluate the boxer's mental alertness, thus screening out preexisting pathologies such as illicit drug usage or neurologic deficit. It also relaxes the boxer to realize that the physician is present as a friend, reducing some of the intimidation that might obstruct useful communication.

The examination of head, eye, ear, nose, and throat should include ophthalmic and fundoscopic evaluation. Palpate the face to be sure that no facial or nasal fractures are present. Grossly examine hearing by rubbing the fingertips near each ear to rule out existing tympanic membrane ruptures. Neck range of motion should be painless and complete. The shoulder, elbow, and hand can be quickly evaluated by moving them through quick ranges of motion and by squeezing the boxer's hands in order to elicit tenderness from any concurrent bone, joint, or tendon injury. A thorough chest exam includes pressing on the rib cage to check for rib pain. The abdominal exam is done to discover enlarged abdominal organs, abdominal tenderness, or masses. The heart and lung exam remains important. A thorough physician evaluating an elite-level boxer competing in a recent National Championship discovered a persistent bradycardia that was confirmed by EKG to demonstrate a second-degree heart block. A check for hernia or testicular mass can be performed on new boxers. A quick observation of heel and toe walking will indicate proper balance and function, while a deep squat should rule out any gross knee, hip, or ankle immobility. Many modifications can be substituted based on the physician's personal preference, as the purpose of this exam remains to prevent preexisting abnormalities from compromising the athlete's safety and performance in the ring.

Ringside Responsibilities

The ringside physician is responsible for seeing that the necessary medical equipment is available and for observing the fight to limit the extent of injuries, to enter the ring to stop the fight or to evaluate the fighters as necessary, and to evaluate the severity of cuts occurring during the bout.

Ringside Supplies: In addition to the usual medical emergency equipment, the physician should have available a small flashlight, gauze sponges, an oral airway, and disposable gloves. These items are frequently needed during the course of competition.

An overlooked supply item that could help in controlling bumps and bruises is readily accessible ice. If the organizers of the event can supply small plastic bags, concession stands usually are willing to provide free access to ice.

Ringside Observation: Each boxer should be intensely observed and studied by the ringside physician during the bout. In fact, as the gong halts the final exchange of punches, an experienced ringside physician should have already mentally imaged what he expects to confirm outside the ring. Skilled observation implies a concentrated viewing of each competitor's actions-reactions, style, skill, offense-defense, and level of activity. Between rounds, clues to injury are enhanced by the busy telltale activities of attending coach and trainer. Their demeanor and priorities serve as blatant directives for our medical concerns.

An active, alert, and focused boxer is not only unhurt, but will probably remain healthy. A hesitant, indecisive, frustrated opponent is likely to be defeated shortly. These roles evolve quite visibly during a bout and serve as an early alert for the referee and doctor. When a boxer is ineffectively defending himself the bout should be stopped. As McCown stated, "A one-sided contest should be halted minutes early, rather than seconds late" (29; p. 76).

Where do we gaze as we monitor a boxer? Sense the alertness in his eyes. Should they become glazed or distant, an examination is warranted. Lowered arms that no longer protect the athlete certainly signal impending trouble. One can monitor a boxer by simply watching his movement; as much can be learned from the feet as from the head. Crisp, balanced footwork assures an alert athlete. A slow, wide-based stance indicates an accumulation of head blows or inferior conditioning and should not be allowed to progress to blatant staggering.

A post-bout exam should most usually be a confirmation of your evolving observational suspicions. However, be open to surprise!

Guidelines for Entering the Ring: Physicians should enter the ring under the following circumstances (30):

1. The referee requests the physician's aid for any serious injury or for an unconscious boxer.
2. The referee requests the physician's evaluation following a standing 8-count.
3. The physician, at his own discretion, indicates to the referee that he wants to examine a boxer between rounds. The referee then signals stop at the beginning of the next round and escorts the boxer to ringside for the physician's evaluation.
4. The physician, at his own discretion, suspends the bout at any time by mounting the ring apron. He should not try to gain the referee's attention by hand signals or by throwing the towel into the ring, but rather mount the ring apron and ask the timekeeper to ring the bell. If the physician thinks that the contestant is in danger of further physical injury, he notifies the referee to terminate the bout at that time. This decision (the ultimate safety of the boxer) takes precedence over all other considerations.

When entering the ring, follow these tips:

1. Enter quickly, but calmly and with authority. Remember, no one else in the ring is as sophisticated medically, and others may tend to become overly excited. Take sterile gauze pads and a penlight with you, and have airway and resuscitation equipment readily available.
2. Do not permit any of the boxers, coaches, or corner personnel to dictate your evaluation. Take all the time you need to evaluate properly.
3. Be sure the boxer has an adequate airway and remove the mouthpiece, watching for aspiration should the boxer be unconscious. If the boxer is unconscious, check for associated cervical spinal injury. If the boxer was knocked to the canvas, insist that he lie down until your evaluation is complete and it is safe for him to come to the sitting position. Only after he is sitting and stable in that position should he be allowed to walk to the corner.
4. When the patient is cleared, he may walk with assistance to the corner and sit on the stool, where further evaluation can continue. After the bout, an injured boxer must be more thoroughly and completely evaluated. This establishes a baseline neurologic exam for further reference should conditions worsen.
5. If a boxer's recovery does not progress rapidly, expedite transfer via stretcher and ambulance (with appropriate neck support) to a

hospital with which arrangements have been made in advance. If recovery from a head blow progresses satisfactorily without evidence of a progressive intracranial process, the boxer is released to the care of his coach or family. The supervising family should be given a head injury slip and thorough explanation of precautions.

6. Give injured boxers a plan for future medical referral and injury follow-up.

A physician should not allow the bout to commence, despite all external pressures, until all safety considerations for that competition have been met. Not too long ago, the senior author was requested to provide medical coverage for a Golden Gloves State Championship Finals. The tournament organizers had failed to make appropriate arrangements with ambulance/ first aid personnel. No first aid personnel, oxygen, stretchers, or evacuation vehicles were present on the premises when the bout was to commence. As a responsible physician, I refused to participate in the event until appropriate contingencies were met. Despite the presence of a large paying audience and local dignitaries, the state championship bouts commenced two hours later than the scheduled starting time of 7:30 p.m. Despite an increasingly hostile audience, we announced in a very positive manner that our paramount concern was the safety of the amateur boxers. Following our message, order was restored and the crowd calmed down and supported our concerns. A negative was turned into a positive!

Evaluating Cuts at Ringside: Occasionally cuts will have to be attended to at ringside. Keep in mind that the boxers, coaches, and crowd may become unnerved by a small cut that bleeds out of proportion to its medical severity.

Figure 7.4 shows facial areas that may be cut during a bout. Around the eye, the presence of any cut that causes enough bleeding to impair vision means the bout should be stopped. Cuts in location A may cause problems with vision and may damage underlying structures. Cuts in location B (the supraorbital nerve) or location C may extend to the nasal lachrymal duct or infraorbital nerve and should indicate cessation of the bout. Cuts in location D, on the upper eyelid, might cause damage to the tarsal plate, which also indicates a need to stop the bout. Vertical cuts at location E through the vermilion border of the lip should stop the bout because of the potential for further tearing of the lip from subsequent blows. Cuts in location F around the bridge of the nose must be carefully checked for evidence of compound nasal fracture. For any cut, if it is obvious that it will not pass a subsequent precompetition exam, the bout should be stopped.

A physician should expect to see small pinpoint oral abrasions in the mouth of the boxer, commonly evident as he spits into the corner bucket between rounds. These nonproblematic oral abrasions are routine and rarely create problems.

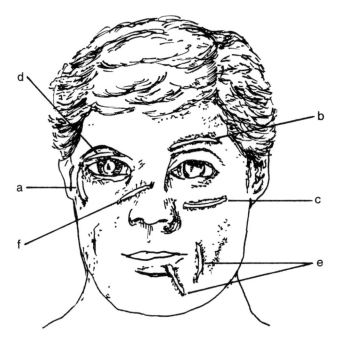

Art by Cathy King

Figure 7.4 Facial areas that may be cut during a bout.
From *USA/ABF Safety Awareness Manual* (p. 56) by USA/ABF, 1988, Colorado Springs: USA/ABF. Copyright 1988 by USA/ABF. Reprinted by permission.

In amateur boxing events, collodion is the only dressing allowed over cuts and epinephrine may not be used as a coagulant. The physician, referee, and trainers should use rubber gloves in the evaluation of cuts, and proper AIDS precautions should prevail.

Post-Bout Examination

Each boxer must be examined after his bout. This process is smoothed by preplanning the pathway of the boxers with the referee, who directs them toward the neutral corner of the examining physician. Forethought prevents chasing the boxers around the gymnasium after their triumphant win or humiliating defeat; their celebration or mourning can commence after the physical examination.

We have been occasionally frustrated by the uncooperative poor loser with an unsupportive coach who refused examination. For the boxer's safety, any unrecognized injuries must be identified. Cooperation can be assured by simply declaring any uncooperative boxer disoriented, thus imposing a 30-day medical suspension (official USA Boxing rule

#107.1[d][ii] [31]). This penalty quickly humbles the arrogant and assures full cooperation.

The post-bout exam requires very little time. As the physician quickly checks pupil reflexes with the light, he can simultaneously look for cuts about the face and mouth. Palpate the face and nose for any area of tenderness, squeeze the ribs, and grip the hands. Even the most stoic athlete will wince as the hands are squeezed when a fracture is present. One need not delay the athlete very long in the post-bout exam if he is appropriately alert and was punching and defending alertly throughout the bout. Any suspicion of injury can be reconfirmed once the athlete has showered and collected himself. Often between current rounds I will recheck an athlete from a prior bout. Seriously injured competitors should be referred to the local hospital, while lesser problems should be monitored according to good instructions provided to a responsible coach or family member.

Traveling Team Physician's Responsibilities (32)

The traveling team doctor's responsibilities include care for the medical needs of the entire delegation during foreign trips. The delegation may include athletes, referees, coaches, trainers, wives, managers, and the doctor. It must be remembered that the athletes and referees cannot be given any substance that will affect judgment or alter their ability to compete. Choosing medications includes considering the risks in the geographic area that will be visited, such as intestinal parasites or poor sanitation. It is recommended that the medication be carried in plastic containers with tamper-proof tops. See that each has a label naming the medication and stating that it is to be used for the boxing delegation. This is particularly important for any narcotics.

Strict adherence will lessen the likelihood of problems with customs authorities at the time of entrance into or departure from each country. It is also advised that the doctor transport copies of his medical and narcotic licenses, as well as any other appropriate medical documents. Recommendations for diagnostic equipment and medications to carry can be found in Figures 7.5 and 7.6, respectively.

Conclusion

The aim of this chapter is to detail the duties and responsibilities of the physician involved with amateur boxing. Adequate care of the boxer is accomplished only with a thorough and comprehensive plan, beginning with a preparticipation examination and ending with a post-bout evaluation. It is the sincere hope of the authors that this chapter will help to maximize safety and promote enjoyment by assisting health care professionals in the care of these talented competitors.

Diagnostic

Ophthalmoscope
Otoscope
Small flashlight or penlight
Stethoscope
Sphygmomanometer
Thermometer
Nasal speculum

Instruments

Disposable suture kits
Forceps
"New Skin" or collodion
Scissors
Steri-strips
Sutures
Scalpels (disposable)
Sterile gloves
Nonsterile gloves
(A sterile suture kit is preferred. Disposable kits are available and acceptable.)

Orthopedic

Finger splints
Adhesive tape

Ace bandage
Soft neck collar
(An ankle splint is handy to have, but not necessary.)

Miscellaneous

Betadine and/or alcohol sponges
Syringes
Needles
Anesthetic (local), Xylocaine 1% or 2%
Airways, at least one large, one medium (adolescent size)
Oral screw
Tongue depressors
Dressings
Eye patch
Band-Aids
Gauze sponge (4 × 4)
Roll-type gauze or Kling
Cotton tip applicators, sterile and nonsterile
Razors (Boxers must be clean shaven)
Plastic Ziploc bags (for ice bags)

Figure 7.5 Items to carry on trips outside of the United States.
From *USA/ABF Safety Awareness Manual* (pp. 57-58) by USA/ABF, 1988, Colorado Springs: USA/ABF. Copyright 1988 by USA/ABF. Reprinted by permission.

1. **Analgesics**—Tylenol, oral and injectable narcotics (minimize). Narcotics should be safeguarded. Aspirin is not recommended just prior to or after a bout because of its anticoagulant effects.
2. **Antihistamines**—Straight antihistamines are not banned, but decongestants (Ephedrine and derivatives) are banned. Oxymetozoline (Afrin) nasal sprays are acceptable.
3. **Antiasthma**—Medication (e.g., Albuterol inhaler). Epinephrine is banned.
4. **Anticonvulsants**
5. **Antibiotics**—For wounds, upper respiratory tract infections, and gastrointestinal infections.
6. **Antidiarrheal**—Imodium is most effective and safe. Caution: Do not use 4 hours prior to bout.
7. **Antacids and antiflatulants**
8. **Antiemetics**
9. **Topical antifungal and antibacterial ointments**
10. **Antitussive**—Dextromethorphan products are accepted for use if drug testing is planned.
11. **Hemorrhoidal**—Suppositories or cream.
12. **Soporifics and sedatives**—Halcion (0.125) is acceptable for sleep, and Benadryl is probably safest; Diazepam-type tranquilizers are acceptable.
13. **Muscle relaxants**
14. **Eye preparations**
15. **Ear preparations**
16. **Laxatives**
17. **Diuretics**—These drugs are banned for use in making weight.
18. **Anti-inflammatory medication**—Ibuprofen, Piroxicam.

Figure 7.6 Medications for travel outside the United States.
From *USA/ABF Safety Awareness Manual* (p. 58) by USA/ABF, 1988, Colorado Springs: USA/ABF. Copyright 1988 by USA/ABF. Adapted by permission.

Acknowledgments

Thanks go to the following people:

Robert P. Nirschl, MD, Virginia Sportsmedicine Institute (Dr. Nirschl assisted in writing the musculoskeletal examination);

Robert Voy, MD, Former Chief Medical Officer of the U.S. Olympic Committee, Las Vegas, NE;

Terry Dusenberry, President of USA Boxing, Portland, OR;

Marilyn Boltano, MD, U.S. Navy, assigned to Walter Reed Hospital, Washington, DC;

Robert Opplinger, PhD, University of Iowa, Iowa City, IA.

The opinions or assertions contained herein are the private views of the authors and are not to be construed as official or as reflecting the views of the Army or the Department of Defense.

References

1. Committee on Medical Aspects of Sports. Statement on boxing. JAMA 181:158; 1962.
2. Morrison, R.G. Medical and public health aspects of boxing. JAMA 255:2475-2480; 1986.
3. Enzenauer, R.W.; Enzenauer, R.J. Boxing-related injuries in the US Army, 1980 through 1985. JAMA 261:1463-1466; 1989.
4. Sammons, J.T. Why physicians should oppose boxing: an inter-disciplinary history perspective. JAMA 261:1484-1486; 1989.
5. Committee on Sports Medicine. Participation in boxing among children and young adults. Pediatrics 74:311-312; 1984.
6. Lundberg, G.D. Boxing should be banned in civilized countries. JAMA 249:250; 1983.
7. Lundberg, G.D. Boxing should be banned in civilized countries— round 2. JAMA 251:2696-2697; 1984.
8. Lundberg, G.D. Boxing should be banned in civilized countries— round 3. JAMA 255:2483-2485; 1986.
9. Richards, N.Y. Boxing: the intent is wrong. Va. Med. 112:122-123; 1985.
10. Proceedings of the House of Delegates, 38th Interim Meeting; 1984, Dec. 2-5. Chicago: American Medical Association; 1984.
11. Jordan, B.D. Medical and safety reforms in boxing. J. Nat. Med. Assoc. 80:407-412; 1988.
12. USA Amateur Boxing Federation. The physician's ringside manual. Colorado Springs: USA Amateur Boxing Federation; 1986.
13. Birrer, R.B. Common sports injuries in youngsters. Oradell, NJ: Medical Economics Co.; 1987.
14. Birrer, R.B.; Wilkerson, L.A. Monographs 71;72-Sports Medicine I/II. Kansas City, MO: American Academy of Family Physicians; 1985.
15. Lane, R.M. Maine code of medical qualifications for participants in interscholastic athletics. J. Maine Med. Assoc. 60:245-254; 1969.
16. Birrer, R.B. Sports medicine for the primary care physician. East Norwalk, CT: Appleton-Centry-Crofts; 1984.
17. Tucker, J.B.; Marron, J.T. The qualification/disqualification process in athletics. Am. Fam. Phy. 40:149-154; 1986.
18. Delp, M.H.; Manning, R.T. Major's physical diagnosis. 9th ed. Philadelphia: WB Saunders Co.; 1981.
19. Mukerji, B.; Alpert, M.A.; Mukerji, V. Cardiovascular changes in athletes. Am. Fam. Phy. 40:169-175; 1989.
20. Maron, B.J.; Roberts, W.C.; McAllister, H.A.; Rosing, D.R.; Epstein, S.E. Sudden death in young athletes. Circulation 62:218-219; 1980.
21. Maron, B.J.; Gaffney, F.A.; Jeresaty, R.M.; McKenna, W.J.; Miller, W.W. Task force #3: Hypertrophic cardiomyopathy, other myopericardium diseases and mitral valve prolapse. Am. J. Cardiol. 6:1215-1217; 1985.

22. American Medical Association, Committee on Medical Aspects of Sports and Committee on Exercise and Physical Fitness. Convulsive disorders and participation in sports. Chicago: AMA; 1969.
23. Shaffer, T.E. The health examination for participation sports. Pediatr. Ann. 7:27-40; 1978.
24. Strong, W.B.; Linder, C.W. Preparticipation health evaluation for competitive sports. Pediatr. Rev. 4:113-122; 1982.
25. American Academy of Pediatrics, Committee on Sports Medicine. Recommendations for participation in competitive sports. Pediatrics. 81:731-738; 1988.
26. Clayton, M.L.; Hamilin, C.; Lewis M.D. Football: the pre-season examination. J. Sports Med. 1:19-24; 1973.
27. Hirsh, P.J.; Hirsch, S.A. Checkout for the would-be athlete. Emerg. Med. 7:65-79; 1980.
28. Lombardo, J.A.; Robinson, J.B.; Smith, D.M. Preparticipation evaluation. Kansas City, MO: American Academy of Family Physicians; 1992.
29. McCown, I.A. Boxing safety and injuries. Phy. Sportsmed. 7:75-82; 1979.
30. Sports Medicine Committee, USA/Amateur Boxing Federation. Ringside physician's certification manual—Guidelines for entering the ring. Colorado Springs: USA/Amateur Boxing Federation; 1990.
31. USA Boxing. Official rules USA Boxing 1993-1995. Colorado Springs: USA Boxing.
32. Sports Medicine Committee, USA/Amateur Boxing Federation. Ringside physician's certification manual—Team physician's responsibility. Colorado Springs: USA/Amateur Boxing Federation; 1990.

BOXING AND SOCIETY

What are the ethical and social implications of boxing in our society? These are the questions addressed in Part III.

The ethics of the existence of boxing are addressed in chapter 8 by Dr. Wildes, an ordained Catholic priest who also has a continuing interest in boxing. He leads us through his argument against the banning of boxing, which holds that, although boxing involves the intentional harming of others, the government has no right to ban the sport because we are a morally pluralistic society with no common moral culture.

In the other chapter of this section, chapter 9, we gain a sociological view of boxing direct from the inside. Dr. Wacquant, the author of this chapter, spent three years in a Chicago ghetto training as an amateur boxer. During that time he learned about the boxers' way of life first-hand, and he interviewed many boxers to understand how they view themselves and boxing. His account gives a clear picture of the pros and cons of boxing for those in lower socioeconomic positions, adding another voice to the debate regarding the value of boxing to society.

CHAPTER **8**

Is Boxing Ethically Supportable?

Kevin W. Wildes

The history of boxing has been surrounded by medical and moral contro-versy. In 1913 a New York court upheld the judgment of the New York State Athletic Commission that Robert Fitzsimmons was unfit to fight and that to allow him to do so would cause serious injury to the man, the sport, *and society* (emphasis added, 1). This judgment was not merely a medical judgment. It also implied a moral judgment, as it asserted a position about what is harmful to society.

Some contemporary historians and critics of boxing have noted that the debate about boxing has now come full circle (2). Jeffrey Sammons argues that the contemporary debate about boxing is not just about the medical aspects of the sport but its moral and sociological status as well. Thus, he thinks the debate has come full circle in that we recognize the harm of boxing as a harm to society. But to "come full circle" means to return to the same place. This is what cannot happen, and this is why the moral argument that calls for government to ban boxing fails. In this century Western society has become morally pluralistic; it no longer shares a common moral culture or content-full moral language. A content-full moral view is one that holds a commitment to a set of values and a ranking of those values. The moral narrative that once shaped Western culture is no longer whole. Multicultural and post-Christian contemporary Western society lacks the capacity for common moral discourse because there are many different moral views and no way in a secular society to know which is correct. This moral pluralism limits the moral justifications that a government can deploy in using coercive power to restrict the liberty of its citizens.

The controversies about boxing and its relationship to medicine provide powerful examples of the crisis for moral thinking in contemporary Western society. The argument that is usually put forward by those who seek to ban boxing is that boxing intentionally causes debilitating medical harms to boxers. These injuries are not side effects of the sport (as in football) but the directly intended effects of the sport. Such behavior, according to this view, is uncivilized and immoral (2-5) and should be banned. Those who argue this position conclude by calling for the state to deploy its coercive power to end the sport of boxing.

The argument against boxing fails. In a morally pluralistic society there are differing views of what constitutes uncivilized and immoral behavior, and there is no universal moral narrative that allows society to make such an evaluation of boxing. People make their own moral evaluations but do so from within particular moral narratives and viewpoints. Each day men and women make judgments about what is morally appropriate or opprobrious. The contemporary crisis for ethics is that Western society no longer shares a common moral narrative that shapes and informs moral judgment (6). Without a shared moral framework there will be different understandings of how boxing should be evaluated and physicians should behave. This problem is evidenced in other moral issues such as abortion or assisted suicide. Furthermore, without a shared, common framework there is no moral justification for the state to use its coercive power to ban activities as long as those who participate do so with free consent.

The first section of this chapter will examine the different ways closure can be reached in moral controversies. The second section will examine the various appeals to moral rationality that have been used in Western culture and the reasons for their failure to provide a foundation for a general secular[1] account of morality. This section is important since it helps make clear why moral controversies are so intractable and why the moral authority of the state is so limited. The third section will examine the implications of moral pluralism for the practice of medicine and boxing.

Reaching Closure in Moral Controversies

Moral controversies emerge when men and women differ on either the description or resolution of a moral dilemma. For some the introduction of the abortifacient drug RU-486 represents a serious moral issue for public debate, whereas for others a ban on RU-486 is the real moral issue. The debate over boxing also illustrates this conceptual problem. The lack of a shared description indicates why moral controversies are often so intractable (8). In part this is so because people frequently hold commitments to different sets of moral values or different views of moral reason.

They cannot even agree on the premises of the argument. Such foundational disagreements often underlie the moral controversies in health care. The controversies over abortion, assisted suicide, and the just distribution of health care resources illustrate such disagreements.

One's understanding of moral reason directs the way in which one thinks about justifying a moral choice (e.g., appeals to rules, principles, virtues, cases) and the values that give content to the reasoning process. As long as men and women share the same understanding of moral reason and moral values, they can, in principle, argue about a moral controversy and reach resolution. Roman Catholics, for example, share a moral tradition that enables them to analyze issues such as professional boxing and understand why the Church would see it as immoral (9, 10). They are an example of a community that possesses a common moral tradition allowing its members to identify moral controversies and acceptable resolutions of them. When men and women have enough moral premises in common, they can reach closure by sound argument (11). However, in a secular, morally pluralistic society, such background assumptions generally are not shared. Thus, this type of closure is not possible.

Moral controversies can also be resolved when consensus is achieved (11). Here it does not matter whether the claims endorsed by the consensus are true or false. All that matters is that there is agreement. In many controversies in health care the achievement of consensus has been sufficient for the resolution of moral controversies (e.g., the national commission to investigate research on human subjects, the president's commission to study bioethics). There are, however, several difficulties with this type of closure.

First, there is often a failure to distinguish between the achievement of consensus and knowledge that it is morally appropriate. For example, the existence of a consensus that hereditary slavery was morally acceptable did not make the practice correct. A consensus indicates that people agree, but it does not indicate the depth of the agreement or whether the agreement is correct. A second difficulty is that while consensus may help resolve a particular case so that the principals (e.g., a physician and patient) reach agreement on what should be done, the adequacy of the consensus may be limited to the particular case. For example, a consensus to limit treatment in one case does not automatically generalize to other cases or into institutional policy on limits to treatment. Finally, it is difficult to understand what role consensus should play in the resolution of moral controversies at the level of public policy disputes in health care (12). In particular, in public policy debates, consensus often does not mean agreement of all parties but the emergence of a majority able to enforce its moral views. The consensus of a moral majority can command no privileged status in a limited democracy. The fact that a majority of people view something as wrong does not mean that it is wrong or that the state should prohibit the activity. Since there is no way, in general secular terms, to know what the correct view is, there is no moral justification for the state to prohibit such activities.

Another sense of closure for moral controversies results from "natural death." That is, a controversy dies because interest in it simply goes away (11). Such closure rarely happens in the moral controversies of bioethics. For example, while the moral controversies that initially surrounded the use of advanced directives have "died," there is continuing controversy about what processes ought to be allowed in the use of such directives (e.g., feeding and hydration, assisted suicide).

There are other ways to close a moral controversy, and these deserve careful examination. Closure can come to a moral controversy by negotiation and appeal to procedures (11). I will argue that the only resolution of secular moral controversies that can be justified to men and women who hold different moral views is an appeal to a procedural morality. That is, since men and women will speak different moral languages and hold different moral views, they will not have enough in common to recognize a content-full closure of a controversy. Yet they may be able to recognize whether there is proper moral authority to close a moral controversy. If one cannot resolve moral controversies by a general consensus, one may decide either to abide by some procedure to create an answer or to apply procedures that draw authority from the permission of those involved. This is why the practice of free and informed consent has come to play such a significant role in health care. If people are in fundamental disagreement about what is proper, they can still act together with a moral authority grounded in their limited agreements. However, to understand why procedural morality has become central to the resolution of moral controversies it is important to review why reason cannot establish a content-full general, secular morality.

The Appeal to Reason

Bioethics has tried to resolve controversies by appeal to sound argument or a set of normative principles or cases. To understand why the only closure possible in a morally pluralistic society is a procedural closure, one must understand why the appeal to arguments, principles, or cases inevitably fails.

The appeal to rationality seems at first to be especially promising. If one is able to provide a definitive rational account of a moral issue, this should resolve all the rational questions advanced by rational individuals. In short, rational individuals could not protest a definitive rational answer to a rational question without declaring their irrationality. Moreover, if one imposes a definitive rational solution on those who rejected it, this imposition would not be untrue to the real nature of those individuals as rational beings. After all, insofar as humans are rational animals, one would realize their true nature by the imposition. The appeal to rationality comes with great promise.

This approach to closure of moral controversies has been central to Western culture since Plato and Socrates. It has deep historical roots in the natural law tradition of the West. Roman law, while acknowledging the practices and customs of different cultures, was shaped under the influences of Cicero, Ulpianus, and Justinian, by a belief in the *jus naturale*, which was known to all animals, and the *jus gentium*, which embodies what reason commands of any rational agent. Gaius speaks of "the law that natural reason establishes among all mankind [and which] is followed by all people alike, and is called *ius gentium* [law of nations or law of the world]" (13; p. 13). This point is repeated in the *Institutes of Justinian* (14). One of the roles of the state was to enforce the moral law. Centuries later, William Blackstone picked up this same theme when he wrote that one of the purposes of the law is supporting the moral law common to all (15). More recently, Lord Patrick Devlin argued that the state should "compel a man to act for his own good" (16). Such views of morality and law obviously form background assumptions for those who desire governments to ban boxing. They argue that the state should act for the good of the individual as well as the good of society. Their argument moves beyond a medical assessment to assert a position about proper behavior.

The hope of a common moral culture was realized in the Christianization of the West. The fabric of faith, culture, and state was symbolically woven together in the crowning of Charlemagne on Christmas Day in A.D. 800 by Pope Leo III. This union of throne and altar symbolized the marriage of the moral law and the civil law. The belief that the moral law could be discovered through natural reason and codified in the civil order became embedded in the Christian view of the world. "God" became the keystone of an ordered, rational universe. After the collapse of the Middle Ages' synthesis of faith and reason, the modern age attempted to provide rational justification for Judeo-Christian morality without faith in the Judeo-Christian God (17). Indeed, the hope of developing a rational, content-full moral theory became the hallmark of the Enlightenment and Western culture (8).

The fundamental conceptual difficulty for the project of resolving moral controversies on the basis of rational argument is that one needs a shared set and ranking of moral values in order to give content to the argument. Such standards have been sought in the following:

1. The very content of ethical claims, or in intuitions, as self-evidently right
2. The consequences of actions
3. The idea of an unbiased choice made by an ideal rational observer or group of rational contractors
4. The idea of rational moral choice itself
5. The nature of reality

None of these strategies can, however, succeed because there is no way to select or discover without controversy the right or true moral content in reason, intuitions, or consequences, or in the world.

• Intuitions. The appeal to intuitions fails because for any one intuition advanced, a contrary one can be advanced with equal ease. The same can be said with regard to compositions or systems of intuitions. What for one individual will appear to be a corrupt or deviant moral intuition can for another appear correct, wholesome, and self-evident. For some, for example, assisted suicide is a horrible sin, while others will think that it is often noble. Boxing will be viewed as "uncivilized" by some and as "sport" by others. There is no way to sort out and rank the intuitions without begging the question and assuming what one seeks to prove.

• Consequences of actions. The appeal to consequences faces the problem of how to assess and evaluate different consequences. For some, living a while longer after chemotherapy is a better consequence, even with side effects, than dying. For others, however, living a life unimpaired by treatment is a more important outcome than extending the quantity of life. To make the judgment one needs a way to rank the different outcomes. A consequentialist will have to build in some presuppositions about the ranking of values in order to evaluate possible outcomes and determine which outcomes are more important and which preferences are to be given priority. One might agree, for example, that the proper goals of political life include liberty, equality, prosperity, and security. Though people may be in agreement with regard to these major goals, one cannot assess consequences until one has decided how to rank or weigh the goals. Different rankings will give decidedly different outcomes; how one ranks the goals will determine whether one is to live in Cambridge or Singapore. Consequentialist accounts are no better advantaged than intuitionist accounts in their ability to demonstrate which set of outcomes is to be preferred, as such a judgment requires an authoritative means of ranking benefits and harms.

The conceptual problem for a general secular morality is that there is no way to discover a ranking of harms. Clearly the critics of boxing see the medical outcomes as harmful and avoidable. However, others may fully understand the medical risks and choose to engage in the sport in the hope of achieving other outcomes (e.g., money, fame, personal satisfaction). Just as with patients who must situate medical benefits and harms within the narratives of their lives, so boxers must do the same. Without having God's view of the universe there is no way for a general, secular morality to rank one set of outcomes over another. We are left in the position that one way of weighing consequences can always be countered by another way of weighing consequences, with no method of judging between them except by appeal to our own moral sense.

• Unbiased choice. Some have attempted to develop content-full, authoritative moral conclusions by employing some variety of hypothetical-choice theory. In such theories an Ideal Observer, or set of choosers, needs to be informed of the various possible choices and to be impartial in weighing everyone's interests and siding with none of the parties involved. But if the observer is truly impartial, how will decisions be made? The observer cannot be so impartial or dispassionate as not to favor certain outcomes over others. Therefore, despite the guide of impartiality, proponents of hypothetical-choice theories must build into the observer some particular moral sense or thin theory of the good (a theory that makes as few assumptions as possible) in the order of choice. As with the intuitionist approach or the consequentialist approach, one needs a way to rank the choices.

One can see this in John Rawls' *A Theory of Justice* (18). By imposing particular constraints on his hypothetical contractors, Rawls builds into his contractors a particular moral sense. They must (1) rank liberty more highly than other societal goods; (2) be risk aversive; (3) not be moved by envy; and (4) be heads of families or be concerned about the members of the next generation. Again the problem is that the description of the contractors presupposes a particular moral point of view. But one is given no independent reason or reasons that argue for one particular view the contractors hold over any other.

• Rational moral choice. Attempts to discover a concrete view of the good life, or justice through analysis of the concepts themselves, suffer the same difficulty as hypothetical-choice theories. One must know, in advance, which sense of rationality, neutrality, or impartiality to use in choosing among different accounts of the good life, justice, or morality. There is no content-full moral vision that is not itself already a particular moral vision. One cannot choose among alternative moral senses or thin theories of the good without already appealing to a moral sense or thin theory of the good.

• The nature of reality. Finally, one is not able to resolve moral controversies by appealing to the structure of reality or nature. This model is known as an appeal to the natural law. It assumes that nature is morally normative and that there is a moral law in the structure of the world and men and women (19). The difficulties here are twofold. First, in order for the structure of reality to serve as a moral criterion, nature must be shown to be morally normative. But in the absence of some metaphysical account of reality, it will be impossible to conclude whether the structure of reality is accidental or morally significant apart from the concerns of particular persons or groups of persons. This is especially the case with regard to human nature, which appears in scientific terms to be the outcome of spontaneous mutations, selective pressures, genetic drift, and constraints set by laws of physics, chemistry, and biology, as well as the effects of catastrophic events. Human nature is, as such, simply a fact of reality without direct normative significance.

The second difficulty with appeal to nature is that even if one thought that one could find moral significance in human nature, this would be possible only if one already possessed a canonical understanding of nature. Even if one accepts the normativity of nature, the structure of reality is open to many descriptions and interpretations. The natural law appeal, like others, must build in some particular moral sense that determines which description of nature is to be normative. However, we have no rational way to demonstrate that one description of nature should supersede all others.

In spite of its attractiveness and historical importance, the appeal to reason for content-fully resolving moral disputes has been a failure. Unless men and women share a common understanding of the moral world or moral rationality, they will be unable to resolve moral disputes in a content-full way. Even if men and women could agree on a particular theoretical approach such as an appeal to consequences or duties or intuitions, the problem remains of selecting a particular guiding moral content. For instance, does one rank liberty over equality or equality over liberty? In order to produce a secular bioethics that can give content-full guidance, one must already have in hand that which one is seeking to discover, namely, a content-full moral vision. A view from nowhere will not give content-full guidance, because it carries with it no particular ranking or account of values. On the other hand, any particular view presupposes what one needs to secure: guiding moral conduct. Generality is purchased at the price of content; content is purchased at the price of generality. This project of justifying a secular bioethics thus appears impossible. Every argument that will lead to a content-full moral conclusion must start from certain particular assumptions. It is just that they will intractably be at dispute in a secular moral society in which there are communities with different moral visions, moral senses, and moral narratives.

Moral Authority

The need for moral authority is real, and it will not go away. To bind together a large-scale society with general moral authority when citizens are members of diverse religious, ideological, and moral communities, one must be able to justify an account of ethics that transcends differences of faith or ideology. Too often secular ethics have simply announced a particular moral view in much the same way that religious visions announce such views. A successful secular ethics must not simply announce a particular moral vision. It must allow diverse ideological visions to have their place (7).

If one cannot appeal to a particular view of morality, there is only one source remaining in which to ground moral authority: the authority of moral agents. If one cannot discover an authoritative moral vision in which to ground moral judgments, then one must appeal to persons as the source of moral authority. When persons meet outside a particular understanding of morality, they have only each other to whom to appeal in order to resolve moral controversies and form public policy. This is the reason for the salience of such practices as free and informed consent, the free market, and limited democracy (with rights to privacy). Absent agreement on external moral standards, the only moral standards possible in a secular world are those derived from the agreement of persons as moral agents.[2]

If one is interested in resolving issues peaceably, without recourse to force and with moral authority that can be understood in general, secular terms, then moral authority can be derived only from the agreement of persons as moral agents. The necessary condition of mutual respect (the nonuse of others without their consent) is integral to a general, secular morality. A morality for moral strangers (those who do not share the same content-full views of morality) requires one not only to refrain from using others without their consent, but also to acknowledge them as agents who can agree or refuse to collaborate.

This basic principle of permission allows us to understand in general secular terms when force and coercion can be justified. Moral strangers may use one another only when they act with conveyed moral authority (permission). Those who use others without consent lose a basis for protest when they are met with punitive or defensive force. Limited democracies draw upon the morality of mutual self-respect to provide protection from and punishment for unconsented-to use of persons (e.g., rape, murder, burglary), as well as to secure the enforcement of contracts.

To face these conceptual problems, the moral authority of the government must be redefined. Absent a common moral vision, the justifiable role of the state becomes minimal. The state has the authority to administer commonly held resources, enforce contracts, and punish those who use others without permission. But it does not have the authority to ban behavior that some, perhaps even many, find morally offensive.

Conclusions

The argument against boxing that is regularly advanced is embedded in a particular view of the moral world. The argument can be structured as follows:

1. Boxing involves the intentional harming of another.
2. Such harms are morally objectionable in a civilized society.
3. As we are a civilized society, boxing should be banned.

The conceptual problem for the argument is that for the argument to be persuasive, there must be a shared view of the moral life that articulates what a morally civilized society is. However, since there is no canonical account of what constitutes a morally acceptable "civilization," the argument will not be compelling in general secular terms. Indeed, in a society that celebrates multiculturalism there are many different accounts of civilization, and no criteria by which to know which account is the best one. While men and women may find boxing morally objectionable, there will be no general secular argument that can justify the use of state authority to ban such activity.

This conceptual dilemma, illustrated by boxing, affects our very understanding of the practice of medicine itself. Health is not only an empirical concept but also a moral one, as it is situated within one's view of what constitutes a good life or a good death. In a society with many views of the good life there will be no single account of the proper moral conduct of medicine. Some physicians, for example, will willingly provide abortions or assist in suicides, while others will vigorously oppose such practices. In such a morally diverse society it is often the case that men and women must tolerate actions they find morally opprobrious (20).

In the midst of such moral diversity, medical practice is marked by the moral authority of both patients and physicians. Patients convey moral authority to physicians so that they may act. Medical practice is built upon a web of agreements between physicians and patients.

Physicians involved in the sport of boxing have the same basic obligations to boxers that they have to their other patients. As with other patients, physicians need to advise fighters of their medical good. However, only the boxer can incorporate the medical good into the narrative of his own life, just as all patients make choices about their medical care with the information given to them by their physicians. As with other patients, physicians retain the right to sign off on a case when they find the choices of their patients to be morally objectionable. One can easily imagine a situation in which a boxer's desire to keep fighting presents, in the physician's judgment, a real medical risk to the long-term health of the boxer. Just as a boxer is free to follow his own conscience, so too the physician must be free. No one can be compelled to act against his or her own moral commitments.

The moral controversy surrounding boxing illustrates not the immorality of boxing, as many think, but rather the conceptual problems for grounding moral authority in a secular society. The controversy makes clear that in a morally pluralistic society the use of state authority to regulate human behavior will be limited. The controversy also illustrates why medicine must be practiced in a web of permissions that give physicians and health care workers the moral authority to act.

Ironically, the debate over boxing and medicine illustrates the inability of general secular ethics to develop a content-full view of this or most other moral controversies. Rather than come full circle, the moral debate over boxing has been entirely changed. Those who would have the state coercively act to ban the sport have not realized that their arguments cannot succeed within general secular discussions in a society that is morally pluralistic. Absent the consent of moral agents, there is a risk of tyranny by those who would impose a particular moral view on others. Those who would have the government ban boxing open the door for the state to act without moral justification in regulating the lives of its citizens.

Notes

[1]The term secular means, at its root, "worldly." It has a long history in which it has been deployed in a number of ways. In this essay I use the term to refer to a neutral framework in which different views of morality come together (see reference 7).

[2]The author of this paper holds that objective standards of morality do exist. The conceptual difficulty for secular moral philosophy is epistemological. There is no "view from nowhere" to enable us to know, by reason alone, which are the correct standards.

References

1. *Fitzsimmons v. New York State Athletic Commission*, 146 NYS 117 (1914).
2. Sammons, J.T. Why physicians should oppose boxing: an interdisciplinary history perspective. JAMA 261:1484-1486; 1989.
3. Lundberg, G. Boxing should be banned in civilized countries. JAMA 249:250; 1983.
4. Lundberg, G. Boxing should be banned in civilized countries—round 2. JAMA 251:2696-2698; 1984.
5. Lundberg, G. Boxing should be banned in civilized countries—round 3. JAMA 255:2483-2485; 1986.
6. Lyotard, J. The postmodern condition: a report on knowledge. Minneapolis: University of Minnesota Press; 1984.
7. Englehardt, H.T. Bioethics and secular humanism: the search for a common morality. Philadelphia: Trinity Press; 1991.
8. MacIntyre, A. After virtue. Notre Dame, IN: University of Notre Dame Press; 1981.
9. Pius XII. Allocution of Italian sporting association, May 20, 1945. In: The Monks of Solesmes, ed. Papal teachings on the human body. Boston: Daughters of St. Paul; 1960: p. 70-78.
10. Davis, H. Moral and pastoral theology: a summary. New York: Sheed and Ward; 1952.

11. Beauchamp, T. Ethical theory and the problem of closure. In: Englehardt, H.T., Jr.; Caplan, A.L., eds. Scientific controversies. Cambridge: Cambridge Univ. Press; 1987: p. 27-48.
12. Bayertz, K. Consensus. Dordrecht, The Netherlands: Kluwer Academic Publishers; 1994.
13. Gaius. Institutes of Gaius. London: Oxford Univ. Press; 1976. Translated from the Latin by de Zulueta.
14. Justinian. Institutes of Justinian. Westport, CT: Greenwood Press; 1922. Translated from the Latin by T. Sandars.
15. Blackstone, W. Blackstone's commentaries. New York: August M. Kelley; 1969.
16. Devlin, P. The enforcement of morals. London: Oxford Univ. Press; 1965.
17. Englehardt, H.T. The foundations of bioethics. New York: Oxford Univ. Press; 1986.
18. Rawls, J. A theory of justice. Cambridge: Belknap Press of Harvard Univ.; 1971.
19. Finnis, J. Fundamentals of ethics. Washington: Georgetown Univ. Press; 1983.
20. Wildes, K.W. Institutional integrity: approval, toleration, and holy war or always true to you in my fashion. J. Med. Philos. 16:211-220; 1991.

CHAPTER 9

Through the Fighter's Eyes: Boxing as a Moral and Sensual World*

Loïc J.D. Wacquant

Man, the sports commentators an' the writers and stuff, they don't know nuthin' abou' the boxin' game. *They ignorant.* I be embarrassed to let somebody hear me say somethin' like that, or write somethin', or print somethin' like tha'. (chuckles in disbelief) "Boxing teach you violence" . . . Tha's showin' *their* ignorance. For one thin', they lookin' at it from a spectator point of view. You know, like seein' a singer an' stuff: he's out dere singin' his butt off an' we lookin' at it 'cause we spectators an' stuff. We his fans, but we don't know when he's out dere, when he's up on the stage, how he—we on the *outsi' lookin' in*, but he's *insi' lookin' out.*

Black lightweight, 28, part-time janitor, 7 years in the ring

In the clamor of opinions that erupt periodically to puzzle out with unfailing fervor and righteousness the perennial question of the anomaly

---

*This chapter is adapted from "The Pugilistic Point of View: How Boxers Think and Feel About Their Trade" by Loïc J.D. Wacquant, 1994, *Theory and Society*, **23**, pp. 902-908, by permission of the editors and Kluwer Academic Publishers.

that the existence of professional boxing seems to constitute in a presumedly civilized society—its (im)morality, the brutality it exemplifies and displays, the exploitation it thrives on, and the destruction in spells[1]—one voice is invariably drowned out and lost: that of the fighters themselves.

The debate swirling about the manly art thus typically turns on the concerns of outsiders to the game, such as the reasons why people should not box, as opposed to the *reasons why they do*—or, to formulate it more rigorously, the pathways through which they come to perceive and experience pugilism as a meaningful avocation to take up and a viable career to pursue. It focuses on the negative determinants, from economic deprivation and school failure to family disorganization and social isolation, that allegedly funnel *lower-class youths* into the ring by constricting other options, and it neglects the *positive attractions* that the trade exerts on its members. It authoritatively imputes a host of individual motivations to boxers, such as a thirst for material success, worldly anger, or masculine pride, but it seldom inquires into the *collective dispositions* that find in this odd craft a public theater of expression and incline some young men from working-class backgrounds to devote themselves to it (Wacquant, 1993).

Testimony about boxing, whether for or against, is characteristically gleaned from the pronouncements of champions, past and present, famous and infamous, as dutifully filtered and refurbished by journalists and sports writers. Occasionally one hears the views of the elite of the coaching corps or those proffered with resounding conceit by top promoters and managers, chief profiteers of this callous commerce of dreams and pain that is professional prizefighting.[2] Only by exception do visions of the manly art issue from the mouths of the rank and file, the "preliminary" boxers, club fighters, prospects and contenders, journeymen and opponents, and trial horses and bums who compose the overwhelming majority

---

[1]"Professional boxing is a throwback, a vestige of our dark, irrational past. That's one reason it is usually under sharp attack in a society that likes to believe it has evolved very different and superior values. You surely cannot reason people into an appreciation of boxing" (Toperoff, 1987, p. 185).

[2]The "insider" literature on boxing is voluminous and comes in a great variety of genres, shapes, and shades, of which only a small sample can be given here. For a selection of the views of three celebrated boxers, see Barrow and Munder (1988) on Joe Louis, Ali and Durham (1975) on Muhammad Ali, and Toperoff (1987) on Sugar Ray Leonard. A revealing collection of interviews of "old timers" from the trainer's guild is that of Fried (1991). For an archtypical expression of the litero-journalistic viewpoint consult Liebling's (1982) vastly overrated *The Sweet Science*; a less pretentious and more perceptive ringside account is Wiley's (1989). Another angle, but always with a focus on the glamour world of elite fighters, is provided by the "ring doctor" Ferdie Pacheco (1992). The experiences of a leading matchmaker are chronicled in Brenner and Nagler (1981).

of practitioners and without whom the boxing economy would instantly collapse, even though they share only its crumbs.

The present article breaks with this externalist, top-down, individualistic perspective on the Sweet Science by taking seriously what ordinary boxers have to say about their occupation: how they think and feel about this harsh craft to which they are willing to give so much, what virtues it holds for them, and how it affects their lives and selves. It highlights selected facets of prizefighting from the "inside looking out," as my gym mate Curtis puts it in the quotation beginning this chapter, in an effort to capture the *positive moment of pugilism*, that spelled by craft, sensuality, and morality. Yet this paper is emphatically not, appearances to the contrary, premised simply on an empathetic "thick description" of the lived experience of prizefighting, an interpretive dissection of "the native's point of view," to recall the words of Bronislaw Malinowski made famous by Clifford Geertz.[3] Rather, it is a (re)construction of the "pugilistic point of view," that is, the synthetic view of professional boxing one can gain from the various points that may be occupied in the structure of social and symbolic relations that make up the pugilistic field. As such, it involves, necessarily, "analyzing the symbolic forms—words, images, institutions, behaviors—in terms of which [boxers] actually represent themselves to themselves and to one another" (Geertz, 1979, p. 228) but it does so firmly on the basis of knowledge of (i) the objective shape of that structure, (ii) its location in the wider social spaces of the ghetto and the city, and (iii) the social trajectory and dispositions of those who enter and compete in it.[4] In short, the ensuing sociological hermeneutic of the boxer's *Lebenswelt* is informed, and rendered possible, by prior recognition of the specific social necessity that inhabits his professional universe.

Adopting the (constructed) standpoint of the fighter, this analysis seeks, however imperfectly, to convey something of the passion, in the double

---

[3]At minimum, it is questionable, first, whether one can pinpoint a single, generic "native" point of view, as opposed to a range of discrepant, competing, or warring viewpoints, depending on structural location within the world under examination. Second, one may query whether the so-called native may be said to have a "point of view" at all, rather than being one with the universe of which she partakes. And third, one must seriously ask whether such a point of view, if it exists, can be explicated: ethnomethodologists have argued, rather forcefully, that such a project is internally contradictory in that it implies treating as a "perspective," a set of perceptual events, precisely what members experience as inherent, necessary, and therefore (at least partly) imperceptible features of their extant environment (Bittner, 1973; Emerson, 1981). My criticism here is more that "thick descriptions" are, as a rule, disembedded reconstructions by the analyst that do not fully recognize themselves as such.

[4]For a terse yet exemplary illustration of this mode of analysis, see Bourdieu's (1988) construction of "Flaubert's Point of View."

sense of love and suffering (the etymological meaning of *patio passus*), that ties boxers to their trade by explicating what it is that they find—or make—desirable and worthwhile about it.[5] For there is a *romance of pugilism* that cannot be elucidated on the basis of the putative financial benefits of prizefighting. Given how little money most fighters earn and the multifold privations they must endure in the monastic day-to-day preparation for fleeting moments of glory or agony in the squared circle, material payoffs come woefully short of accounting for the seductions of boxing. To understand what drives fighters—their quasi-sacrificial giving of themselves to their occupation—one must heed and disclose the latter's moral and sensual attractions.[6]

This paper is based on a large body of observational, life-story, documentary, and experiential data produced in the course of an ethnographic study of the social world of professional boxers in the black ghetto of Chicago. From August of 1988 until October of 1991 I trained and hung out regularly at the Stoneland Boys Club, a "traditionalist" boxing gym located on a dilapidated stretch of one of the main thoroughfares of the city's South Side.[7] There I not only learned the craft and took part in all phases and aspects of the boxer's Spartan regimen;[8] I also socialized and evolved solid friendships with a number of fighters, trainers, managers, and other "fight people" whom I followed in their daily round. This long

---

[5] I use the erotic (or psychoanalytic) notion of "desire" advisedly here because, as will be seen below, these bonds of love have deep-seated sensual (and sexual) roots and they are inseparable from the production and validation of a public (hyper)masculine self that is one of the immaterial yet very real personal profits of boxing. I say that boxers (also) "make" boxing desirable to emphasize that the process under analysis is not a passive one of "reception " but, rather, entails an infinite series of microscopic, mostly unreflective, acts of appropriation of the extant social world and the possibilities it offers to those endowed with the proper categories of perception, appreciation, and action.

[6] This effort parallels that of Jack Katz (1989) as he unearths the sensual and moral attractions of criminal activity in his germinal book *The Seductions of Crime*. Katz showed how explanations of criminal violence remain incomplete so long as they fail to unravel its experiential foreground and dynamics.

[7] The atmosphere and mode of functioning of professional boxing gyms varies with the personality, pedagogic style, and authority of their head coach, and secondarily as a function of their ethnic recruitment and status in the local or national boxing economy. Stoneland's gym (a pseudonym) was directed by a world-reputed trainer "from the old school" who tolerated few if any violations of the "sanctity of immemorial traditions" (Weber) as handed down by predecessors. It thus offered an ideal site for vivisecting the culture and economy of prizefighting.

[8] I started literally from scratch, with no knowledge of the game and precious little "raw talent." Indeed, I was so awkward and incompetent at first that Shante, a

period of immersion allowed me to observe boxers and their entourage in their natural habitat and to experience firsthand the process of inculcation of the pugilistic *illusio*—the half-inarticulate, quasi-organismic belief in the value of the game and its stakes, inscribed deep within the body through progressive in-corporation of its core tenets. I was also in a position to trace out the economic, cultural, and moral roots of boxing as a (sub)proletarian bodily trade providing a supplement or an alternative to more conventional avenues of livelihood and mobility such as the school, the low-wage labor market, and the informal street economy of the ghetto.[9]

In this tentative and partial sketch of the pugilistic point of view, I draw especially on in-depth, semistructured interviews with 50 fighters (36 Afro-Americans, 6 Latinos, and 8 whites) comprising nearly all of the professionals active in the state of Illinois during the summer of 1991. These face-to-face interviews, typically lasting close to two hours and yielding some 1,800 pages of printed transcripts, were conducted in settings ranging from boxing gyms and automobiles to local diners to the residence of the boxer or investigator.[10] They are complemented by, and interpreted in the light of, extensive notes from my field diary as well as information culled from innumerable informal conversations in gymnasia, at weigh-ins, or during or after boxing shows throughout the Chicago metropolitan area or on the road, as well as in the neighborhoods and homes of my fighter friends. Because I had been part of the local landscape for almost three years at the time of formal interviewing and had proven my genuine interest in the game by "paying my dues" in the ring, I could establish a relation of trust and mutual respect with the boxers. Because I had by then become fully conversant with their cultural idiom, I was able to phrase my questions in a manner congruent with their occupational

---

rising welterweight unbeaten in ten straight fights who would later become my closest friend and sparring partner, used to ask the coach when I would train to come take in the hilarious spectacle of ineptitude I was offering daily from the back of the gym. But with tenacity, dedication, and the sage pedagogic guidance of the gym's veteran head trainer, I eventually improved enough to spar on a regular basis with "pros" and to compete in the 1990 Chicago Golden Gloves tournament. I also worked as a trainer's assistant and generally observed up close all facets of the game, from dieting, refereeing, and weigh-ins to contract negotiations with managers and transactions with promoters.

[9]See Wacquant (1992a) for a fuller discussion of the method and data used in this study and Wacquant (1994a) for a sociological picture of the surrounding ghetto.

[10] Two of them were done by telephone due to intractable problems of transportation and scheduling. Several were prolonged by follow-up interviews and informal conversations (most often in the gym) that were taped, transcribed, and appended to the original interview.

concerns and thus elicit candid and meaningful answers. Finally, my extensive firsthand and scholarly knowledge of the daily tribulations of boxers in the ghetto allowed me to probe and check (or triangulate) these answers and to elaborate a variety of leads so as to get as close as possible to the fighter's lived understanding of his trade.[11] Having established myself as a member (albeit of a marginal sort) of the guild, then, was the basis of my ability to develop an "intuitive and provisional representation of the generative formula of each specific interviewee" (Bourdieu, 1993, p. 911), just as it was critical in enabling me to get interviewees to cooperate in unveiling this formula more fully so as to pinpoint its invariants.[12]

One last prefatory qualification is in order. For reasons of analytic strategy (and lack of space), this paper deliberately brackets the objective factors and material forces that bear upon the lifeworld of professional boxers and give it its peculiar structure and feel. It does not address the broader matrix of class inequality, caste exclusion, and plebeian masculinity that continually replenishes the supply of fighters and the asymmetric system of positions and transactions that define the division of labor

---

[11]At the same time, such an endeavor comes up against a well-nigh irresolvable problem: how to communicate with words, on paper, in an intellectually coherent and intersubjectively resonant manner, an experience that is as profoundly organismic, sensual, and submerged beneath (or is it beyond?) the level of discourse as prizefighting? There can be no satisfactory resolution of this question, only practical attempts at answering it. Yet to reduce it to a mere problem of "poetics" (as recent "postmodern" anthropology has been wont to do, cf. Clifford, 1991) and to propose a rhetorical remedy—say, to concoct a melange of representational strategies mixing realist, surrealist, and impressionistic tropes in a "dialogical" or polyphonous key—is to miss the real issue, which is: Are there not things about human social practice that we understand as practitioners, through "carnal knowledge," that we cannot communicate in a scholarly (or scholastic) idiom, through the mediation of symbols? And if so, what are we to do with them?

[12]In about a third of the cases, these interviews, coming at the end of three years of intense "observant participation," were not the product of a fleeting and superficial encounter but one link in an extended chain of routine interpersonal exchanges. Even those boxers and trainers who did not know me personally when I approached them at this stage were aware of my "insider status" and could situate me on the local pugilistic scene ("Yeah, I seen you at fights, you one of [coach] DeeDee's boys"). Any other approach would have generated enormous distortions likely to mutilate, if not destroy, the object to be constructed, through a combination of diffidence, self-mystifying miscommunication, and deliberate mythologizing. For a discussion of friendship as a necessary social condition for the production of nonartifactual ethnographic data in oppressive social settings such as the black American ghetto, see Wacquant (1994d).

undergirding this "political meat market"[13] that is the boxing business. Thus it remains, on the face of it, agnostic as to whether the views and beliefs of pugilists are ultimately beneficial to them or to what degree they partake instead of a "collective self-deception," to invoke Marcel Mauss's formulation, to which boxers are both unwitting participants and consenting victims.

This question, whose resolution is here postponed, is not a mere analytical conundrum—and its evocation a discursive gesture of complicity aimed at those social theorists concerned with the fashionable puzzle of "structure and agency" or submission and resistance. It is one that tugs at the kernel of the pugilistic cosmos and tears, however furtively, at the soul of each of its inhabitants. As adumbrated in the concluding section, prizefighting is a social universe riddled with ambivalence, a turbid, double-sided, Janus-faced world suffused by dubiety and suspicion even as it trumpets its certitude and proclaims its time-honored truths with an air of unbendable defiance.

Fighting the Trope of Violence

Boxin' doesn't jus' teach you violence. I think, boxin' teaches you discipline an' self-respect an' it's also teachin' you how to defen' yourself, so, it's really great to box. It's a lot of fun. Anybody who feels that it teaches you violence is a person tha's really a, a *real incompetent mind* I think. Someone tha' their min's thinkin' real low.

Kenny, black middleweight, 24, night security guard, 8 years in the ring

If there is a single set of recurrent images and narrative strategies—what Arjun Appadurai (1988) calls, in another context, a "strong trope"—that dominates the public representation of boxing, it is no doubt that of violence: The unmediated, unbridled fistic onslaught of man upon man is unquestionably the most graphic picture spontaneously associated with prizefighting. Savage blows hurled to the head of a defenseless combatant, blood squirting from mouth and nose, cut eyebrows and shattered bones, battered bodies crumpled in pain on a stained ring mat as the crowd clamors for more: Even people who have never set foot in a gym or

---

[13]Expressions drawn from the occupational lingo of professional pugilism are placed in quotation marks. Emphases in the interview excerpts are those of the boxers unless otherwise indicated. Names and other identifying characteristics have been altered or removed whenever necessary to protect the privacy of informants.

witnessed a live fight are well acquainted with these visions.[14] From a distance, boxing resembles nothing more than a miniature realization of Hobbes' state of nature, a"warre of every man against every man," a brutish clash of bodies governed by "force and fraud."

This common perception is not without grounds. Of all combat sports, boxing is, along with wrestling, the one in which physical confrontation is the least aestheticized and euphemized. As a "percussion sport" involving direct, agonistic corporeal contact, pugilism distinguishes itself sharply from "prehension sports" such as judo in terms of both means and ends (Clément, 1987): Competition in the ring aims not at thwarting or coralling the moves of the opponent but at delivering potent blows to his head and upper body so as to inflict superior physical damage and, if possible, render him incapable or unwilling to sustain the contest.[15] The total subordination of form to function that turns the body into the weapon and target of deliberate assault inevitably results in real physical erosion that is amply documented by biomedical studies of boxing (e.g., Morrison, 1986). Injuries and bodily deterioration are not incidental to the game; they are the necessary outcome of proper professional exertion. One plays basketball and even football; one does not "play" at boxing. As my old coach phrases it: "Ain't no such thing as 'recreational boxing,' Louie. You get in d'ring, this is serious biz'ness: somebody's up in there tryin' to tear your head off."

Boxing is a true "blood sport" in ways that few if any other athletic activities are, as reflected in the hypermasculine ethos that underpins it. The fistic trade puts a high premium on physical toughness and the ability to withstand—as well as dish out—pain and bodily harm. The *specific honor* of the pugilist, like that of the ancient gladiator, consists in refusing to concede and kneel down. One of the visible signs of that much-revered quality called "heart" said to epitomize the authentic boxer is the capacity not to bow under pressure, to "suck it up" and keep on fighting, no matter what the physical toll.[16] A pug who quits in the midst of battle is

---

[14] The main source of this surface familiarity today is the complacent (and wildly exaggerated) staging of gory scenes of ring demolition in countless motion pictures, of which Sylvester Stallone's fictionalized fistic heroics in the *Rocky* series is one particularly popular exemplar.

[15] When he was asked during testimony before a congressional commission if he knew he had Jimmy Doyle in trouble during their 1947 fight, which ended tragically with Doyle dying from the sequelae of a brutal knockout, Sugar Ray Robinson could only answer in his equanimously gentle voice: "Sir, they pay me to get them in trouble" (in Wiley, 1989, p. 121).

[16] Much like the drama of *pankration*, one of its premodern ancestors in ancient Greece, boxing turns on the "ostentatious display of the warrior virtues" (Elias & Dunning, 1986, p. 138): "Victory or defeat was in the hands of the gods. What

branded with the mark of infamy and suffers a veritable symbolic death. Accordingly, the occupational idiolect of boxing gives pride of place to military expressions and metaphors: Valiant fighters are "gladiators" who go to "war," throw "bombs" at each other, and exhibit "ring generalship" in implementing their "search and destroy mission."

Last, there is no denying that the intimate familiarity with violence that comes with growing up in a poor urban neighborhood rife with crime constitutes good preliminary preparation for the ring in that it raises one's threshold of tolerance for belligerence and inclines one to a radically instrumentalist conception of the body well suited to professional pugilism.[17] My coach was quick to detect such qualities as a means to estimate the future ring potential of a novice:

> I stayed late for this new guy last night but, boy, was it worth it! . . . He real tough, *he been shot, he been stabbed three times*, so he tough, he can take pain awright. He been in jail, tha's where he learn to box. Then he stop for two year but he fight on d'street. He aggressive, he's quick. He got bad balance but he can hit you, *boy he can hit*! Anybody he hit with a right hand, he gonna put'em away, knock'em cold as a milkshake.

Yet to equate pugilism with physical aggression *tout court*—as historian Jeffrey Sammons (1988) does when he writes that the very existence of boxing "reflects society's fear of and need for violence"—is a distortion bordering on disfigurement in that it arbitrarily reduces a multifaceted bodily occupation to only *one* of its aspects—and to one especially salient and objectionable to nonparticipants. It contradicts, nay defiles, the lived experience of fighters who disagree forcefully and unanimously with the idea that boxing is a school of brutality.[18] Indeed, many can scarcely

---

was inglorious and shameful was to surrender victory without a sufficient show of bravery and endurance." After noting that former title holder Hector "Macho Man" Camacho "took so much punishment in his 12-round points loss to Chavez in September 1992 that he is probably finished as a serious contender," the boxing newsletter *Flash* commends him for showing "the grit of a champion in surviving [the bout] by never going down" (*Flash*, 131, December 20, 1993, p. 3).

[17] I showed elsewhere that boxers view their body as a weapon, a tool, and a machine, in short, as the specific capital and instrument of labor they invest in the pugilistic economy (Wacquant, 1994a).

[18] Only 6% of Chicago fighters concede that "all that boxing teaches you is violence, how to beat up another man." A comrade from Stoneland's gym exclaims: "Those are *ignorant people*! Those are ignorant people! Put that in your book Louie." And a seasoned Latino welterweight who once had a taste of the "big time" in Las Vegas explains the halo effect that associates boxing with unruliness and aggression: "I know where you git it from, lotta guys that are boxers, professional fighters and

contain their indignation at such a notion and retort that it testifies to the ignorance and disrespect of those who hold it. "It's mostly probably people who have nothin' to do with the sport that would probably think that it's a violent sport," reflects Roy, a black middleweight who gave up a stable job as a cable installer for a suburban television company to devote himself full time to his fistic calling. "They don't look at the aspect where it's *keepin' youth*, young men *off the street*. It's a way to *benefit* yourself if you're *not* in college or you don't have a great payin' job—if you can fight, if you're good with your hands, it's a way to success, too."

The suggestion that boxing should be banned because it is brutal strikes fighters as both incongruous and hypocritical. Why single out sport from a myriad of activities and objects that are considerably more destructive, yet fully legal and quite commonplace, such as guns, automobiles, or the consumption of addictive substances?[19] "I think we should protest," elaborates Eddie, one of the trainers at the Stoneland Boys Club. "I say if we close down the gym, let's close down the liquor stores, also. Let's close down the lounges also, 'cause that creates a lotta violence. I say: *don't stress on one point*." And why in addition unfairly single out boxing of all sports? Fighters correctly point out that their trade is no more violent than other, more "mainstream" athletic pursuits that have captured the fancy of the American public, such as football, in which high rates of both chronic and acute injury are quite normal,[20] and even basketball ("Basketball has gotten very physical right now, that is the winnin' right

---

they git in trouble ba-ba-bah, but mosta time, lotta the boxing guys, they come from (derogatory tone) *ghettos, proje'ts* and all the, y'know, they're in *gangs*, ba-ba-bah. They're like, Mike Tyson, okay? For example, Mike Tyson: why is he the way he is? 'Cause he was brought up that way, *right*? He was on the street, is it because he boxes? No, he was like that, tha's how it is with a lot of these guys."

[19]Dean, a former fighter and referee who runs an amateur gym in one of the city's Chicano barrios, rails: "Boxing, *it saves lives*, it saves lives (a tad exasperated at the question). If you're going to ban something, (forcefully, each tirade gushing forth with increasing conviction) *ban alcohol, ban cigarettes, you know, ban coffee*—I'm a drug addict, I gotta have a cup of coffee in the morning. You know, ban that stuff. That's worse for you, you know, especially cigarettes! Jeez, what a killer that is! Uh, *ban automobiles*! Uh . . . automobiles kill you, *the fumes, look at what they do to the air*! There is other things they should ban beside boxing, I don't know. No, no, boxing is good for a kid."

[20]Injury is an institutionalized aspect of professional football. "Playing hurt" is a banal, expected, and even publicly valorized (and glamorized) aspect of the game. Every week NFL teams are required to release a "report card" on their health status, including a roster of players in various states of physical disrepair (probable, doubtful, on injured reserved, on non-football injury list, etc.). Injuries routinely suffered in a game include concussions, cuts, torn ligaments, dislocated limbs and joints, deep bruises, and fractures. Unlike boxers, who are automatically

now, through physical play: Look at the Detroit Pistons!''), not to mention stock car racing and more exotic sporting quests such as parachuting and hang gliding. True, one can suffer grievous physical damage, even ruination, in the ring, but as fighters note, ''you can get hurt doin' any-thin' '': one can walk outside and get run over by a car, or get mugged and clobbered to a pulp on the street. The fact is, most boxers reside in segregated and degraded neighborhoods where violent crime is a basic fact of everyday life and where physical insecurity infests all spheres of existence (Wacquant, 1994b). Against the backdrop of such a harsh urban environment, boxing can hardly seem particularly violent.

Pugilists are also quick to underline that anyone who wants to dispense brutality has only to pick up a gun, a knife, a brick, or a baseball bat to be in a position to mete out physical punishment with much greater ease and effect than with gloved fists. Consider the differences—as marked as those ''between night and day,'' my coach was fond of saying—between boxing and street fracas. Fighting in the ring is governed by strict rules, upheld by a neutral authority, that curb the scope and level of aggression and substantially attenuate its impact. Free-style fighting on the street, by contrast, has no clear boundaries regarding location, duration, means, and participants, as Bernard, a black light-heavyweight employed as an x-ray technician in one of the city's most prestigious hospitals, explains:

> Streetfightin', I'll prob'ly, half-*kill* a person. Boxin' is *skill*. You got gloves on your hands an' you can't really kill a person, as quick as you could with your hands. [In streetfighting] you don't have any rules. You can pick a bottle up. You can go home an' get a gun an' come back, you know, or tell a big brother. You know, a frien' coul' jump in an' double-team you. You ha' rules. I don't look at boxin', you know—there's a lot of articles abou' boxin' shoul' be banned an' thin's of tha' nature, but boxin' to me is a sport. It's not tryinna knock, tryinna kill a person, it's jus' tryinna accumulate punches an' beat this guy an' knock him down, but *en route to tha'*, if it gets a lil' more serious, then you have to do what you have to do, but it *is* a sport. It has *rules* and there is a point of sportsmanship involved in boxing. It differs vastly, you know, from street fightin'.

In fact, there are grounds for arguing that boxing does not fuel but rather depresses the level of interpersonal and public violence by channeling

---

suspended for 90 days following a knockout, quarterbacks are known (if not expected) to return to action shortly after being taken off the field due to a concussion (LA Raiders passer Jeff Hoffstettler was celebrated for his bravery after doing so twice in the same game in the fall of 1993).

aggressive impulses within an organized, collective framework that rigidly regulates its display and endows it with structure, purpose, and meaning. First, daily "roadwork" and training in the gym drain the energies out of fighters and likely absorb whatever *Angriffslust* they might hold. "In my opinion, it *relaxes* the fighter that's in you 'cause you releases it an' it just makes you a calm, all-around better person," comments Keith, a quiet, surly 24-year-old welterweight who works part time as a radio station announcer and has not been embroiled in a single street confrontation since signing up at Stoneland. Tony, a truck driver from one of the city's white ethnic neighborhoods who campaigns in the light-heavyweight division, adds:

> It's a *skill*, it's a sport to be better than a person. I don't think violence and all (shakes his head vigorously), I don't agree with that. I tell ya the truth: ever since I started boxing, I've been more of a mellow person. I've been more relaxed. Like I said, I'm not, all my aggressions are taken out. In the gym I work out, I come home, someone come up to me and say "yer an asshole," I'm like, (with a smirk) "you're right!" You know, I'm *mellowed out*. I'm way mellowed out.

One need not subscribe to the "hydraulic" theory of violence according to which (male) human beings have a natural propensity toward aggression, a predetermined quantity of which has to find an outlet somewhere—if not in war, crime, public disorder, and domestic violence, then in combat sports or vicariously through the spectacle of destructiveness in the media[21]—to understand that a young man who gets up at five in the morning to run four miles in the cold and spars eight hard rounds in the afternoon is unlikely to roam the streets at night looking for trouble.[22] Second, by the very nature of their activity, boxers acquire a great deal of personal confidence and a sense of inner assurance that militates against recourse

---

[21]This ancient nostrum has recently been revived and given a new pop-psychological twist by the self-styled advocates of the "mythopoetic men's movement": "If a culture does not deal with the warrior energy . . . it will turn up outside in the form of street gangs, wife beating, drug violence, brutality to children, and aimless murder" (Bly, 1990, p. 38).

[22]According to the trainer-in-second of the Stoneland Boys Club, "when a kid leaves that gym from trainin', he don't feel like doin' anything else: he's tired. He don't have that energy to get out on d'street and stick som'body up or somethin'. He just wanna go home and get some rest." My personal experience confirms this: The most strenuous and anguishing aspect of conducting ethnographic fieldwork among boxers was not to step into the ring to "rumble" but to sit at my personal computer at home upon returning from the gym for hours of note-taking in a half-comatose state of extreme physical and mental exhaustion.

to violence in interpersonal relations. To function in the ring, pugilists must bring their emotions under firm stewardship, vanquish their most intimate fears, and learn to monitor themselves continuously—their physical state and mental moods, their sleep and eating habits, their sexual and romantic involvements, their family and social life—in ways that cannot but increase their feeling of self-mastery (Wacquant, 1994a). A journeyman heavyweight who works as a prison warden and had to overcome a deep streak of timidity to join the brotherhood of Fistiania expresses this view tersely: "When you have confidence, you're not afraid of people, you know, you don't lash out at them, you just—you're secure in yourself, and you don't need to lash out at the world."

Third and more generally, the microcosm of the gym in which fighters spend much of their waking time forms "a vast tissue of reciprocal activity"—to borrow Cooley's (1966) definition of society—that tends to deflect and contain forms of interpersonal bellicosity owing to the norms of civility, fairness, and reciprocity that hold sway within it (Wacquant, 1992a). A properly run boxing gym is one where boxers are required to behave in a courteous and respectful manner toward each other and their entourages and where no fights or scuffles occur outside the ring. If boxers have conflicts and grudges to settle, they are invited to do so between the ropes and according to the rules of the trade (i.e., wearing a head guard, mouthpiece, and heavily padded sparring gloves, and in three-minute rounds). The gym constitutes a *small-scale civilizing machine* in Elias's (1982) sense of the term: It simultaneously imposes strict taboos on certain forms of violence, lowers one's threshold of acceptance of disorderly behavior, and promotes the internalization of controls and obedience to authority. Thus immersion in the "personal community" (Wellman, 1982) formed by the gym membership and broader boxing fraternity tends to reduce the "lust for attacking" that prizefighting appears to exemplify and thrive on.

Last, as will be shown later, pugilists value their technical know-how and the "professional" status that it imparts to them. A central component of the occupational ethic of pugilism, which coaches impress upon their charges from the first stages of initiation on, holds that fistic prowess must be reserved exclusively for display in the ring against properly prepared opponents. It is not to be squandered by unregulated and irregular usage in an improper setting (such as the streets) or debased by being directed at persons untutored in the pugilistic idiom and devoid of skill or strength, and even less so against persons statutorily unfit to respond on an equal footing to a methodical fistic attack, such as women.[23] This is the reason prizefighters (try to) shun street altercations and situations

---

[23]Long after his retirement, "Smokin' " Joe Frazier put the gloves back on to give a good "ass-whuppin' " in the ring to his son and successor Marvin (who later challenged for the world heavyweight title) after he had punched a young woman.

that might require them to come to blows with others. Some will go to extremes to avoid "wild" fights and are even willing to lose face momentarily to prevent a challenge from escalating into a full-blown clash. Others use a "bodyguard"—generally a muscular or heavyset friend or relative— for close personal protection in order to lower the odds of a confrontation in public places. "If somebody tries to pick a fight on the street," advises Ishmael, a Puerto Rican middleweight who toils as a grade man laying asphalt all day before calling to the gym, "you gotta back away, you back away, you can never start a fight, I mean you know, the dude could be cussin' you out, your mother, your daddy, you gotta back away 'cuz you're a registered fighter and you cannot touch 'em, *unless* they lay a hand on you." This is recommended in light of the risk of injury and legal complications that might ensue, but more fundamentally it is a question of professional morality and self-respect.[24]

"A Technician Type of Thang": Pugilism as a Skilled Bodily Craft

Boxin' is like, it's like uh, *electrician.* It's a *skill.* It's a' art. I mean, how many people can take wire an' rewire this whole buildin', an' then you gotta ask yourself how many people can box? It's jus' a skill. It's a plus.

James, black heavyweight, 29, informal day labor, 6 years in the ring

Fighters conceive of boxing not as a springboard for aggression and an exercise in violence but as a skilled bodily trade, a competitive performance craft requiring sophisticated technical know-how and an abiding moral commitment that will enable them not only to improve their material lot but also, and more urgently, to construct a *publicly recognized, heroic self.* Boxing is the vehicle for a project of *ontological transcendence* whereby those who embrace it seek literally to fashion themselves into a new being so as to escape the common determinations that bear upon them and the social insignificance to which these determinations condemn them.

Such is the fundamental paradox of prizefighting: To outsiders it stands as the ultimate form of dispossession and dependency, a vicious and

---

As Marvin recounts it (in Berger, 1993, p. 17), "[He said:] 'I'll teach you what to be sorry for, you sissy'. He got mad. I haven't hit a girl since." Coaches consistently warn their fighters against using their fists on their spouse or lover (which, of course, does not mean that it does not happen). A member of the Stoneland Boys Club was expelled from the gym immediately after a trainer caught him slapping his girlfriend at the back of the building.

[24]Muhammad Ali recalls how he resisted getting drawn into a physical confrontation during a racist incident in a Louisville restaurant shortly after winning the gold medal in the 1960 Olympics: "I had already signed for my first professional bout. It's part of the pride of a truly professional fighter not to indulge himself, not to be caught dead or alive in a free-for-all" (Ali & Durham, 1975, p. 66).

debasing form of submission to external constraints and material necessity. For boxers it represents the potential means for carving out a margin of autonomy from their oppressive circumstances and for expressing their ability to seize their own fate and remake it in accordance with their inner wishes.[25] The ring affords them a rare opportunity—the only one that many of them may ever enjoy—to shape to a degree their own destiny and accede to a socially recognized form of existence. This is why, in spite of all the pain, the suffering, and the ruthless exploitation it entails, of which fighters are vividly aware, boxing can infuse their lives with a sense of value, excitement, and accomplishment.

Prizefighting is first and most evidently a *working-class job*, that is, a means of earning a living or, to be more precise, of augmenting other sources of income[26] by exchanging the only tangible asset that those bereft of inherited wealth and educational credentials possess: their body and the abilities it harbors. "It's a job, tha's how I make my money, tha's how I get paid," avers Aaron, a black lightweight from a northern suburb of Chicago with an undistinguished record of four defeats in six bouts. "Doin' it for money and stuff, it's *like a second job*, like the other guy's a fighter, he's doin' it for money, you're doin' it for money. That's the way I see it," chimes in Ishmael. Drake, a 32-year-old journeyman welterweight who first "gloved up" at age twelve and has accumulated 45 fights in his eleven years as a pro, agrees:

It's somethin' I do jus' to—*I box because it's a payday*, y'know what I mean, I feel then as, you know, how, it put somethin' in my pocket and add *more luxury to my life*, man. I figure, if I get in the ring now, I'm able to do it now *but*, I do it, I does it only 'cause at the moment I *get paid* to do it and it's somethin' I can do and I enjoy doin' it.

---

[25] There is no room here to adequately address the nature and social foundations of this paradox. Suffice it to note that, while they universally denounce the abuse and exploitation to which they are exposed, boxers nearly always deny also that one can be coerced into the ring, and they vigorously claim (at least partial) responsibility for their fate between the ropes, as my sparring partner Shante does when he clamors that "it's up to the fighter to fight, Louie: *cain' nobody make me fight! Cain' nobody make you fight!* You come in there with the understandin' of whatever you know you gonna do. If you ain' prepared, tha's *your fault.*"

[26] Few fighters can survive solely on fight purses, which are very minimal at the club and regional levels: between 150 and 500 dollars on average for preliminary bouts from four to eight rounds, and between 500 and 1,000 dollars for most ten-round "main events" in the Midwest. Nor can they rely exclusively on support from their managers, when they do have one who agrees to pay them a "weekly salary" to train (of, say, 150 dollars per week). Thus a majority of boxers maintain full- or part-time employment as they fight (50% and 12%, respectively, in Illinois).

That boxing is a working-class occupation is reflected not only in the physical nature of the activity but also in the social recruitment of its practitioners and in their continuing dependence on blue-collar or unskilled service jobs to support their career in the ring. It is indicated also by the fact that fighters consider training not as avocation and relaxation but plainly as work: "It's a job before's anything else, an' it's entertainment when you in that ring. But the *trainin's* your job," insists Roy. "Work, work. I'm goin' to work, shovel the dirt: This yo' job," agrees Ned, a colleague from the South Side who is attempting a comeback after a two-year layoff. Yet professional prizefighting differs from, and is deemed preferable to, low-wage labor in several crucial respects.

First, unlike factory jobs, for instance, fighting is a form of physical work that boxers seek out and appreciate because it grants them a high degree of control over the labor process and unparalleled independence from direct supervision. True, the occupational ethic of "sacrifice" demands that they submit to a rigorous regimen of training and to the strict authority of their coach (Wacquant, 1994a), and if they are at all serious about getting ahead in the game, they will also have to bear the tutelage of a manager. But this disciplinary framework is one they consent to by the very fact of entering the trade and one they perceive as ultimately beneficial to them. What is more, it leaves them a good measure of autonomy in designing and executing the daily routines that make up their professional duties. Fighters maintain that they cannot be made to train and fight against their will: They have to desire to be in the ring. Nor do they have interest in "slacking off," given that they are the ones who will suffer the consequences of a lack of dedication and intensity in the ring. Boxers place great value upon being their "own boss" and in claiming accountability for the outcome of their occupational efforts.

Second, although it may not appear as such to the untrained spectator, boxing is a *highly skilled activity* that requires mastery of a complex and multilayered corpus of knowledge.[27] The view that fighting in the ring is a matter of naked strength and raw aggression is a gross misperception, one that Henri, a black light-heavyweight who has fought professionally for over a decade in addition to holding a highly paid job in a chemical factory, is quick to put to rest:[28]

---

[27]Much the same was true of gladiators in ancient Rome, where it was a skilled trade whether or not the public recognized it: "Gladiatorship was not to be reduced to a sordid butchery: it was an art of the sword. Indeed, the military theorist Vegece liked to extol the skills of his gladiators to the soldiers of the legions in order to stimulate them" (Golvin & Landes, 1990, p. 168).

[28] Vincent, a black middleweight who recently moved back to Chicago after a disappointing foray into the West Coast boxing circuit, concurs: "My mentality

It's a *thinkin' man's game*, but the outside doesn't see that. The on'y thin' they see is jus' two guys throwin' punches, you know. Well, uh, you gotta think about *what* you gonna do, *when* you gonna do it and *how* you gonna do it. See, this is what you gotta think about . . . [Through training eventually] it comes natural. When I see you, I know exactly what I got to do. See, I'm always lookin' for the openin', I take what you give me. I always have to beat you from your mistakes.

A well-known gym adage holds that boxing is "seventy-five percent physical and seventy-five percent mental," which is to say that fighting requires not only bodily strength and technical prowess but also moral resolve and tactical intelligence. Because a bout is a quintessentially strategic and interactive contest, mastering the basic punches (jab, hook, cross, uppercuts) and moves (feints and parries, pivots, blocks, and so on) and being versed in the intricacies of ring generalship is far from sufficient. A fighter must also develop the ability to combine and integrate these elements afresh during each bout to resolve the practical conundrum posed by his opponent's repertoire of physical, technical, and tactical tools. Once between the ropes, you must instantaneously identify the strengths and weaknesses of your antagonist, adjust to (or disrupt) his rhythm, and decide, in a matter of a split second, "how you execute punches, when you're gonna do it, what timin' . . . It's not like *two chicken fightin'*," insists Jeff, a 29-year-old white welterweight entering his seventh year as a pro. "I mean you *box* an' you movin' around an' you're thinkin' about what you gotta do an' what you're gonna execute, you know. Double up on your jabs, get the guy goin' backwards or jab, hook off your jab." An Italian-American trainer from a West Side gym elaborates:

It's jus' like when you play like a game, Monopoly or somethin': it's who *outsmarts* the other guy . . . I tell 'em in the ring, it's who's gotta be the better man, you know: you gotta use *strategy*,

---

is that it's a *science, it's a work of art and beauty*: I like to make a man miss, you know, *counter-punch*, show my superiority by speed and skills, not so much by goin' out and say 'I'll just show I'm a stronger brute and more of a *macho man* than you, and jus' beat the hell outa you and bust you up' and things of that nature." And Anthony, a 27-year part-time athletic instructor going into his second year as a pro, puts it this way: "I look at it as a way of life, it's somethin' *to do*, it's somethin' to master, it's a technique of your whole body: see you might master a computer or a calculator, somethin' like that. Well I master how to use my arms as somethin' that was made from scientists or fightin' goin' back to the eighth dynasty—they're the ones that thought up boxin', karate, these arts, so I'm bringin' out what they invent a long time ago an' *masterin' it the proper way*."

sometimes you gotta use *strength*, sometimes you haveta use *move-ment*, you know it's—it's jus' not gettin' in there an' jus' beatin' up the other man, *it's an art*, like dancin', you know: you learn steps, you learn moves, you go through *a lotta* trainin' for it, (gesturing with his hands) you don't jus' come in there an' in three days have a fight.

Much like the work of an electrician, a welder, or a potter (Linhart, 1976; Needleman, 1979), pugilism requires an indexical, context-sensitive, embodied competence that is not amenable to being extracted from its natural setting and grasped outside of the concrete conditions of its actualization. It is a *kinetic technique* consisting of trained physical, cognitive, emotional, and conative dispositions that cannot be handed down or learned via the medium of theory but must instead be practically *implanted*, so to speak, into the fighter through direct embodiment (Wacquant, 1992a, 1992b). This means that it takes years of arduous and intensive training, as well as extensive ring experience, to acquire proper command of the game. Most trainers estimate that a minimum of three to four years are necessary to produce a proficient amateur fighter and an additional three years to mold a competent pro. "There's no short cut in boxin' and learnin' *how* to fight is not easy progress," remarks my old trainer, "Yeah, because you take a hundred guys come in d'gymnasium maybe *two* may become fighters." This in turn helps explain the highly distinctive value of the fistic vocation: Anybody can pick up a job in a factory or peddle drugs on a street corner; not everyone has the mettle to step into the ring and even more so the "spunk" to virtually retire into the gym for years and put up with the unyielding discipline of mind and body this demands.[29] Genuine commitment and love of the game are indispensable to sustain a fighter over time. In this respect, as well as in terms of both autonomy and skill, boxers resemble the artisan more than they do the classical proletarian of Marxian theory: They are small entrepreneurs in risky bodily performance.

Third, unlike most of the low-paying, dead-end, unskilled jobs to which young men from the inner city are being massively relegated in the new urban economy (Sullivan, 1989), boxing offers the *prospect—however illusory—of a career*, that is, the possibility of advancement through a sequence of hierarchically ordered positions on an ascending scale of status, prestige, and income. Even better: For a few, those who somehow succeed in assembling the winning package of heart, talent, and "the right people behind them," it holds out the promise of striking it rich and

---

[29]The veritable social incarceration that boxing requires is admirably rendered in W.C. Heinz's (1984) novel *The Professional*.

escaping once and for all "the life of the urban serf."[30] From unknown club fighter to prospect to contender to champion, every trail of sweat and blood promises to lead to Las Vegas and the "big time," the one "payday" that will make it all worthwhile—and more. Over 80% of active professional fighters in Chicago subscribe to the idea that boxing offers a viable avenue out of poverty. And virtually all of them (upwards of 85%) believe, at least at the outset of their careers, that they have a chance to rise all the way to the top and become world champion.[31] At minimum, and in contradistinction to standard wage labor in which exertion and remuneration are blatantly uncorrelated, boxing promises that persistent effort will ultimately be rewarded: "It's a skill to learn, somethin' in life that you like doin', it's like . . . it's like really like *bein' on a job*, eight hours a day in the gym—an' it pays off, an' it pays off in the long run," assures Matt, a black cruiserweight from the South Side who twice fought for a world title.

Last, and related to the previous point, boxing is a glamorous profession, highly prized not so much by the broader society as by what Tocqueville called the "little society" of relatives, peers, and neighbors. The prestige of the Sweet Science in low-income neighborhoods is based essentially on the fact that it gives a dramatized public expression to the virile values (such as hardness, pugnacity, and physical bravery) that compose the common bedrock of working-class cultures across ethnoracial divides (Horowitz, 1982; Foley, 1990; Connell, 1991).[32] It is reinforced by boxing's association with the wider media-dominated constellation of professional sports, arguably the single most alluring sector of individual achievement today among lower-class youths and, in particular, black youths (Rudman, 1986). The ring could prove to be a springboard to stardom and a bridge

---

[30]As Gerald Early (1991, p. 178) writes of Joe Louis and Sonny Liston: "They understood each other well because they knew the fates they would have suffered had they not become boxers, the fates of working-class men, black and white, who lived anywhere: a life of crime or a life of ordinary manual labor, the life of the urban serf."

[31]To account for this extraordinary figure (few elective professions feed unrealistic career expectations with just this kind of ferocity), one would need to analyze both the structural bases of occupational oneirism (such as the dyadic and intransitive nature of boxing hierarchies, the lability and impermanence of bodily capital, and the corresponding fuzziness of evaluative criteria), the recruiting trajectory of prizefighters (many of whom enter the trade burdened with the disillusion of aborted careers in other sports), and the relentless work of collective mystification necessary to sustain commitment to the game.

[32]A 32-year-old black middleweight from the Stoneland Boys Club with over a decade of ring experience has this comment: "Everybody knows a boxer is a *tough individual* an' anytime you climb in the ring and put yo' life on the line, people

to the enticing, otherworldly universe of VIPs and celebrities (Gamson, 1994). The symbolic capital attached to being a professional athlete is all the easier to appropriate owing to public ignorance of the abysmal differences in earnings and career patterns between "name fighters" and club fighters.[33] Taking their cues from the million-dollar purses they read about in newspaper stories on high-profile—but highly atypical—heavyweight title fights, most people believe that preliminary boxers collect large purses, in the thousands of dollars and more, when in fact they are barely scraping up a few hundred dollars for weeks of onerous preparation. A black welterweight who supports himself by combining boxing with a range of "hustles" on the streets of the South Side ghetto confesses with embarrassment: "It's like [I'm] *a idol*, I got a lotta peoples in my neighborhood, know I'm a good fighter, they wanna idolize me, an' I ain't even makin' no money!"[34]

As several of the foregoing quotes clearly show, the pugilist's conception of his craft is not entirely shorn of an aesthetic dimension. Not, to be sure, in the "highbrow" sense of a detached concern for the expressiveness and coherence of forms and a celebration of their finality; nor even as a "grounded aesthetics" woven into the fabric of personalized acts of cultural consumption (Willis et al., 1990). The boxer's specific sense of beauty resides in a critical and knowing appreciation of the instantaneous strategic mastery of a tangled set of techniques, constraints, and contingencies requiring poise, dexterity, sureness of judgment, and pinpoint accuracy, as well as trenchant intervention towards the attainment of one's goal. Ed, a 36-year-old black cruiserweight who doubles as a correctional

---

pat you on the back because you doin' somethin tha' you coul' win' up gittin' hurt seriously wounded or even murdered, so they give you praise and glory for you to be a warrior like that, go in the ring and come out." His gym mate Ed further expounds: "It is *admired*, I mean, jus' like how folk go to professional fights an' see two fighters step in the ring: there's that fear, that (guttural grunt) '*HUUUN!*', that *awe*, okay?"

[33] This capital is especially high among young lower-class women who, according to boxers, are prone to be impressed by their credentials as "professional athletes," as Vincent relates: "A lotta women won't admit it and so forth, but I think they look at that, you know, you're a fighter because—*first of all, most people are in this fantasy world* that all fighters have a lotta money, or make a lotta money. And then they think that you're the tough guy, the guy they can look to for *protection*, and so forth, and it's like—especially if you're one that's been on television, and so forth, like I was in the Los Angeles area, and it felt like you're walkin' around with a big star or somebody that's on his way."

[34] Another indicator of the adulation that boxers enjoy in their immediate social circle: People often call them "champ" irrespective of their achievement in the ring, or lack thereof. It is the case even of a mediocre 33-year-old black middleweight with only four wins in twelve fights: 'They look up, *it's a good feelin'*

officer and counselor in a halfway house and came to boxing after an abbreviated career in professional football, verbalizes it thus:

> I mean, to be able to stand before a man, a *massive* man, an' he punches you an' he goes through efforts to hit-an'-harm you, an' he's unable to even touch you an' you're no more than uh, (whispering excitedly) twelve inches away from him: that, that, it takes an art to be able to do that. . . . That's to be able to have *your rhythm*, to put forth your own individual *style*, and have it portrayed and presented to the public, uh to be able to, I mean, *have an art*, and have it appreciated, you know: it's very beneficial.

What makes boxing an art for prizefighters is not, as sports writers and scholars contend, that it constitutes a "symbolic dialogue" (Ashworth, 1971) and, even less, a "conversation" that pugilists would hold by way of "their physiques" (Mailer, 1971). It is "the techniques you haveta go through, the trainin' you gotta go through," and the unique fusion of body and mind, instinct and strategy, emotion and rationality that must be demonstrated *in actu*, in the effectual *doings* of combat. Pugilistic beauty resides in the practicalities of the fight itself, not in what it signifies, as the following comment by Jeff makes obvious: "Bein' able to deliver a punch jus' the way you picture it in your head, how you gonna do it, you know: I mean *that's an art.* Jus' the *right timin', the right speed an' everythin'*, it's, (raving) it's a helluva feelin' after you been trainin' all this time an' hit somebody with that perfect punch."

If pugilism may be said to be artistic, then, it is less in the sense of Kant's aesthetics, as an expression of a pure disposition to "differentiate" and "appreciate" beauty rooted in one's inner sensibility, than as a manifestation of what Thorstein Veblen (1948) called the "instinct of workmanship": an interested, this-worldly appreciation of the "efficient use of the means at hand and adequate management of the resources available for the purposes of life."[35] For my gym mate Lorenzo, a 24-year-old welterweight who broke into the world rankings after toiling six years in the amateurs and three years in the pros, fighting is just such "a *technician type of thang*, it's a *beautiful thing to do*, you know: I like to watch

---

because when you're runnin' an' people blow their horns at you, I tell 'em like this, when I'm runnin' they say 'go ahead champ!' or blow, blow the horns: that gives me strength when I'm tired an' that lets me know that I got the support an' it makes me work harder."

[35]"I threw punches with bad intentions . . . I was trying to hit him behind the ear, in a vital area. . . . Did you see that hook? Ooo, that was nice! That took all the fight right out of him" (Mike Tyson, commenting on a knockout victory over heavyweight rival Pinklon Thomas, quoted in Wiley, 1989, p. 187).

tapes of boxers at work." And he goes on to reject the trope of violence and to assert instead the theme of love:

> Everybody, a lotta people look at boxing as a fightin', brutal sport, but you know it's not *that* to me. I done uh seen all the pretty boxers in the world fight you know so to me it's a technician art, you know, it's beautiful boxin'. [There is an aspect of beauty in boxing?] Yeah, I feels it in the ring, that's why I like it, *I love it so much—not like it—I love it* so much exactly. I love what I do.

"An Affectionate Love"; or, the Sensual Rewards of Prizefighting

"You gotta love it. I walk it, talk it, sleep it, act it, look it. Some people don't believe me when I say I'm miserable as hell around the house if I'm not doing anything," once revealed "Marvellous" Marvin Hagler (in Nack, 1982, p. 94). Much the same is true of club fighters and journeymen who will never enjoy a fraction of the wealth and fame attained by the bald-headed middleweight champion. For boxers are bound to their trade by a profound, multifaceted, sensuous relationship of affection and obsessive devotion, an organic connection (*sympatheia*) akin to a religious allegiance inscribed in their whole being—or, better yet, a form of *possession* born of the thorough refashioning of their "lived body" (Merleau-Ponty, 1945) to accord with the specific temporal, physiological, and cognitive-emotional stipulations of the game.[36] Fighting is not simply something that they do, an instrumental activity, a pastime and a side job separable from their persona. Because it demands and effects a far-reaching restructuring of the self as well as an integral colonization of one's lifeworld, boxing is what they *are*: it defines at once their innermost identity, their practical attachments and everyday doings, and their access to and place in the public realm.[37] The reason boxers seem unable to retire from the game on a clean break, submits Vinnie, a white "prospect" who is supported by his manager and has run up eleven victories in a row since his

---

[36]Wiley (1989, p. 158) gives a capsule description of this all-consuming dilection and how it can overwhelm all other pursuits: "Fighting was [world champion Thomas] Hearns' single abiding interest. He bought a Young Chang grand piano and didn't learn to play a single note. He ordered the construction of an ornate bar in his home, but didn't drink. He built a glove-shaped pool, but didn't swim. He talked of becoming a businessman, while talk of business easily bored him. He said he wanted to be an actor, yet his expression never changed. A confirmed bachelor, he drove a gold 500 series Mercedes Benz. But he was not a carouser. He'd rather spar with you than speak with you." Numerous other illustrations could be culled from my ethnographic diary and from the published biographies of champions.

[37]A 30-year-old black heavyweight who has slugged with most of the "big names" of his division in the four years of his professional career summarizes the matter

20th birthday, is "because it becomes *part of their inside*, it becomes part of their *heart*, like you might say, they might wanna quit, they might not wanna come to the gym, (passionately) but it's *always* a part of 'em: *they're a fighter man!*"

Material insecurity and the attendant project of economic betterment can scarcely account for the fervor and depth of the commitment that binds pugilists to their craft. The proof is that few of them would trade their bruising occupation for a secure job in the wage-labor economy, even one that would allow them to provide adequately for themselves and their family.[38] Asked whether they would "hang it up" if they found a "good job" (however they choose to define it), two thirds of the Windy City's pugilists answer negatively. "No, I *love* boxin'," says Dave, a 26-year-old janitor who just turned professional after nine years spent battling in the amateurs. "Boxin' is my first priority, y'know, it's *my life, it's a job for me, it's a career.*" A young black heavyweight from the far South Side entering his third year as a pro echoes:

> *I don't know*, I don't think, it'd have to be a real goo' job. Have to be a real goo' job. Be makin' a lot of money an' havin' a lot of benefits, 'cause *I don't see shit makin' me quit boxing*. I don't see nothin' coul' make me quit boxin' right now. Not even a goo' job. I woul' try to work a goo' job an' *still* box. I like it.

A journeyman lightweight who joined the ranks of the professionals in his early 20s after a mediocre amateur career in the military and aspires to "a job paying fifteen bucks an hour" that would mark a substantial improvement over his current employment situation—he works some 70 hours a week as a carpenter in his brother's shop for scarcely a thousand dollars per month—would not give up the trade for that: "Nope, I *gotta go*: Once you put your mind to somethin', you gotta stick with it, no matter how many bumps you take along the line, you gotta stick it out, you gotta stick it out. We gonna make it."

Pugilists commonly call forth biological metaphors of drugs and contamination to articulate the *visceral infatuation* they nourish for their

---

well: "Why is it that I get in the ring? Because I have been *trained* to get in the ring, an' I have the *heart* to get in the ring, an' it's a part of my *livin'* so I haveta get in the ring, it's somethin' that I *like*, an' always I'm enjoyin' it." Under this angle, boxing may be considered as a form of "identity work" realized not through talk, as in Snow and Anderson's (1987) analysis of the techniques of salvation of the self among the homeless, but through bodily work and performance.

[38]Also, a good many boxers sacrifice immediate occupational opportunity and advancement to their pugilistic ambitions, leaving jobs either because they are physically demanding and consume too much of their energies or because of conflict between their work and training schedules.

occupation and the moral compulsion they feel to give it all that they have. "I wouldn't wanna say it's a disease," ponders Jesse, a 29-year-old Latino policeman who entered the gym at age 14 and has fought almost uninterruptedly since. "I don't think it's a disease, it's jus' an *affectionate love* that I have for boxin'." Fighting, they explain, is "something that's in your blood," that you cannot "get out of your system" once you have had a taste of it, even though it may threaten ultimately to destroy you.[39] Boxers also borrow from the lexicon of romantic love to express the fondness and reverence they hold for the Sweet Science, speaking of the latter as one would of a difficult but sultry lover or, better yet, a voluptuous and feisty mistress who is ever covetous and trying but whose magnetism cannot be forsaken or evaded. "You put in so much of yer time, you know, blood and sweat all them years, you know—how could you jus' walk away from it?" rhetorically asks a 26-year-old white middleweight entering his third year as a pro. "I don't know many people that just *divorced* it an' never looked back, so I think it's too hard."[40]

As with singing, dancing, preaching, and kindred body-centered performance trades that traditionally occupy a pivotal place in working-class culture, especially Afro-American (e.g., Keil, 1966; Allen, 1991; Davis, 1985), pugilistic prowess is considered by many to be a sacred gift, a charismatic skill bestowed by a higher authority whose possession carries with it the moral obligation to cultivate and use it well. Like verbal dexterity in the case of the black preacher, fighters hold that boxing is something that they have "in them" and that it would be unconscionable not to exploit such inner treasure and to fail to realize the destiny it might hold for them. The carnal attraction of pugilism is so potent that boxers can lose their ability to conceive of themselves apart from their ring

---

[39] This happened in a physical sense to boxing's most famed and beloved figure, Muhammad Ali, about whom trainer Angelo Dundee remarked: "Muhammad was never happy outside the ring. He loved boxing. The gym, the competition. It was *in his blood*, and win or lose, he loved it to the end" (in Hauser, 1991, p. 399; emphasis added).

[40] Or, to cite one variation on this theme: "Fighting is like a wife. It can be good to you, if you treat it right. If you don't, then, like a wife it will know, because it's right there with you all the time" (former champion Bobby Chacon, cited by Wiley, 1989, p. 135). Boxing does in many ways constitute a structural counterpart and rival to the pugilist's lover in that it causes a diversion of his time, energies, and mental and emotional investments from the domestic (and erotic) sphere, in effect arrogating to itself the fighter's libido. Revealingly, fighters who "break training" by missing a gym session or by engaging in sexual intercourse before a bout often say that they feel guilty of "cheating," as if boxing was their true life companion.

activity.[41] Indeed, in many cases fighting grows so entangled with their sense of self, so intricately braided into the emotional and mental fabric of their individuality that they simply cannot envision life without it.[42] Says an unemployed black middleweight who migrated to Chicago from a small southern town four years ago to chase his dreams of pugilistic glory:

> I get in the ring, it's more of a, it's a emotional combine with the *skills*, combine with somethin' I wanna do. It's, it's jus' somethin' I like to do, it's make me feel like *I'm me*. It jus' gonna make Willie M—— gittin' in the ring. It make Willie M—— Willie M——. Right now, if I wadden in the ring, Willie M—— woul' ha' to fin' somethin' else to do. Right now, the ring is what make Willie M—— be Willie M——. I feel at home in the ring. I feel like this is *my* environment, this is where it's me. Jus' like them jobs, tha's what I am: I'm a boxer.

Kenny has taken a night job as a security guard to reserve his day for training. He works from eleven to seven the next morning, comes home, sleeps until early afternoon, and then heads out to the gym. He would not have it any other way:

> I love boxin'. I know the fundamentals of the sport, you know, this what makes me happy. If I didn't do this, I *woul'n' be happy, man!* I be out there doin' somethin' wrong. I think I prob'ly *die*, you know, (cheerfully) 'cause it's what I live for, it's jus' a great sport to me. I jus' love doin' it.

Boxers feel that, by stepping into the squared circle, they can achieve something inaccessible or forbidden to them outside, whether it is wealth, fame, excitement, a sense of personal control and moral proficiency, or simply the unspeakable prosaic joys of being caught up in a thickly knit

---

[41]Freud (1962, p. 13) argues in *Civilization and its Discontents* that love is fundamentally an experience of blending that entails an illusory fusion such that "the boundary between ego and object threatens to melt away."

[42]It is this passionate love, more than cool calculations of economic gain, that impels fighters to seek to return to the ring following a life-threatening injury. Rhode Island's Vinnie Pazienza stunned the boxing world—not to mention his neurosurgeons—when he reentered the fray (and went on to win a world championship) only months after having suffered a near-lethal crushing of several vertebrae in his neck during an automobile collision. On the morrow of a brush with death in the ring from a massive brain hematoma that sent him into a coma and left him partially paralyzed, "Kid" Akeem Anifowoshe defiantly announced from his hospital bed that he would again seek a world title: "I want to get myself back as soon as possible. Believe me, I will do anything to fight again. Slow by slow. Take your time. The dream is not over yet" (in Berger, 1993, pp. 39, 19-23).

web of tensionful activities that valorize them and imbue their life with elan, drive, and significance. Most importantly, all these rewards can seemingly be attained under their own powers, as an outcome of their individual choices and strivings, *volens et libens*, thus attesting to their operative faculty to elude the common constraints that limit others around them. In sum, predilection for prizefighting is not so much (or not only) a reaction to material deprivation as a recourse for elaborating, and then responding to, an *existential challenge of one's own making*, under conditions such that the ring appears as the most attractive arena in which to wage it.

Boxing is "where the action is": a universe in which the most minute behavior is "fateful," that is, problematic and highly consequential for the individual engaged in it (Goffman, 1967).[43] By entering an occupation that hinges on "the willful undertaking of serious chances" (Goffman, 1967), boxers decisively realign the structure and texture of their entire existence—its temporal flow, its cognitive and sentient profile, its psychological and social complexion—in ways that put them in a unique position to assert their agency. For with risk comes the possibility of control; with pain and sacrifice, the eventuality of moral elevation and public recognition; and with discipline and commitment, the existential profit of personal renewal and even transcendence. Through the ministry of boxing, fighters strive to remake themselves and the world about them.

Professional pugilism enables its devotees to escape the realm of mundanity and the ontological obscurity to which their undistinguished lives, insecure jobs, and cramped family circumstances relegate them and enter instead into an extraordinary, "hyperreal" space in which a purified and magnified masculine self may be achieved.[44] It does this first by thrusting them in the midst of a *luxuriant sensory landscape*, a broad and varied panorama of affect, pleasure, and dramatic release. By virtue of its closure to the outside and the severe psychophysical regimentation it requires, the pugilistic universe features a unique "tension-balance between emotional control and emotional stimulation" that generates unparalleled excitement and offers ongoing "emotional refreshment" to its participants (Elias & Dunning, 1986). Set against the monochromatic tone of everyday life in the shadow of urban marginality, even the highly reiterative and

---

[43]Goffman (1967, pp. 174, 181) explicitly lists boxing among the "professional spectator sports whose performers place money, reputation, and physical safety in jeopardy at the same time," and which he sees as paradigmatic of "action" (and he cites Arond and Weinberg's famous 1952 sketch of the "occupational subculture of the boxer").

[44]For perceptive accounts of a similar quest in other existential realms, read Katz's (1989) analysis of the "Ways of the Badass" and Fussell's (1992) account of his conversion to the cult of muscularity. For further comparison, see Adler and Adler (1991) on the collective production of the "gloried self" among college basketball players.

predictable routine of training is animated and alluring due to the shift it causes in the "balance of the sensorium" (Synnott, 1993) and to the continual kinesthetic, visual, tactile, and aural stimulation it procures. For the boxer, working out daily is like an interminable journey of exploration across the vast expanses of his corporeal territory. Through endless repetition of the same drills (shadow-boxing, punching an assortment of bags, skipping rope, sparring, and calisthenics), he learns to dialogue with, and monitor, different body parts, striving to expand their sensory and motor powers, extend their tolerance to strain and pain, and coordinate them ever more closely as his organism slowly imbibes the actional and perceptual schemata constitutive of the pugilist's craft. Turning one's body into an impeccably tuned fighting machine is an absorbing and rewarding process in its own right. "When you get outa the gym you feel like a brand new person. Some people like t'get high an' *that's my high,*" muses a Mexican-American middleweight who has spent over a decade patrolling the rings of the Midwest. "That's a great feelin', that you're in shape an' you live a disciplined life, there's nothin' like it in the world—you're *on cloud nine,*" confirms Jeff.

Over the long-winding cycle of emotional "highs and lows" (Steinross & Kleinman, 1989) spanned by weeks of preparation for a bout, boxers weave a delicate tapestry of affective materials mingling anxiety and anger, aggression and fear, impatience and elation. Riding the pugilistic roller coaster gives life a sparkle and zing that it would scarcely have otherwise. Danny, a Puerto Rican cruiserweight with a record of two defeats and two draws for only one victory, discloses that he steps into the ring "to have fun, it's, it's *thrillin': you don't know what's gonna happen in the ring an' I love it. I hate bein' bored with the same thing over an' over. An' the boxin' everytime—I could spar with you ten times an' ten times it will be a different fight.*" And he refers in stride to the so-called greatest upset in boxing history, namely James "Buster" Douglas's stunning knockout of the previously invincible Mike Tyson in Tokyo in the winter of 1990, as proof that anything can happen between the ropes.[45]

The emotional acme of the boxer's life, however, is reached not in training but during the official bout itself—and in the hours and minutes before and after confrontation between the ropes. The fight is a sensory

---

[45]Danny continues: "That is the thing I love about boxin': you never know what's gonna happen, especially with the heavyweight, you never know when that big punch is gonna land. A guy could land it to you, you could land it to them, an' it's like *all over,* you know, in a second an' that excitement that goes in, gives you a rush, that excitement, it's like *'wow!* this is what I want, a little danger." A cogent case for the potency of such "expressive joy" in motivating risky action is Rosaldo's (1989) analysis of the moral-emotional seductions of head-hunting among the Ilongot of Northern Luzon in the Philippines.

microcosm unto itself, characterized by a drastic narrowing of one's sentient receptivity, high-speed processing of stressful stimuli under acute urgency so as to impose order on a complex and entropic perceptual field verging at times on complete chaos, and a virtual merging with the task at hand leading to the euphoric experience of "flow" (Csikszentmihalyi, 1981) and an intense sensation of self-possession. Like other "edgeworkers" such as test pilots, high-speed boat racers, and sky divers (Lyng, 1990), boxers insist that fighting has ineffable qualities that cannot be captured and conveyed linguistically to outsiders. And they doubt that any other pursuit could give them the thrill of fistic battle. You have to experience in your own flesh the coeval anguish and excitment of "going toe-to-toe" as the culminating trial of weeks of taxing training to fully grasp boxing's sensuous magnetism. Marty, a 22-year-old white featherweight who turned pro at 17, recounts the conclusion of his last bout:

> There's no explanation for the feeling you got when there's, y'know, two thousand people screamin' your name, y'know, and you got your hands up. Right then it's just a feeling that, you just can't even *explain*, I mean I get the goosebumps just thinkin' about it! You—you can't explain it. It's *better'n sex for me*, I think. I mean, I, there's nothin' I could even compare it to.

The emotional profile of the postfight phase is no less rugged, mixing ever-fluctuating doses of relief, pride, shame, and joy. Always present, so long as the boxer prepared dutifully and "sacrificed" as prescribed by his profession's ethical code, is a radiating sentiment of personal competency and accomplishment: "Afterwards, win or lose, you know you jus' go an' shake hands an' you compliment the guy that you fought an' it's jus' the *greatest, greatest feeling*," nods Roy. Fighters frequently compare the solace that fills them after a bout to reaching a mountaintop from which they can dive back into the tranquil flow of everyday life and savor the mundane delights they have been foregoing for weeks: watching television late at night, feasting on cheeseburgers and milkshakes, going out and resuming amorous intercourse. One South Side pug compares the feeling to "takin' a safe off your back," another likens it to "gettin' a orgasm," while a third prefers a parallel with celebrating Christmas or a surprise birthday party.[46] One thing that boxing is definitely not for its practitioners is indifferent and dull.

The Morality of Boxing

"The voluntary taking of serious chances is a means for the maintenance and acquisition of character," writes Goffman (1967) in his pioneering

---

[46]Nate, an unemployed black welterweight who has boxed on and off as a professional for five years, voices this sense of accomplishment thus: "Well it's like

analysis of fateful action. A second major immaterial attraction of professional prizefighting is that, being premised on a logic of agonistic challenge and strict obedience to an all-embracing ascetic life plan, it supplies a highly effective procedure for publicly establishing one's fortitude and valor. Between the ropes, one can be proven beyond dispute to be a man of strength (*vir fortis*) but also, and perhaps more importantly, *a man of virtue*. Boxing, it is said amongst the fraternity of pugs, "tells the truth" about a person—and not only about his public and professional side as a ring warrior but about his inner worth as a private individual as well.

The homology set up in and by the ring between physical excellence and moral standing rests first on the idea, enshrined in the ubiquitous notion of "sacrifice," that success in the fistic arena hinges on the adoption of proper personal habits and conduct outside of it. It is believed that an ordinary boxer who conscientiously abides by the commandments of the pugilistic catechism, as they apply in particular to nutrition, social life, and sexual activity, stands every chance of toppling a more talented but dissipated foe: "It's good fighters get beat by guys tha's not good as they are because this man that *did right*, he's the better man," philosophizes Stoneland's old coach.[47] Irrespective of whether such justice prevails in actuality, pugilism is a system of education (*disciplina*) that endows the boxer's life with moral tenor by the simple fact that it enregiments it and submits it to a soldierly discipline exceptional for its extensiveness and austerity.[48]

Second, boxing "tells the truth" because it subjects its practitioners to the probing scrutiny and public judgment of like-minded others, both members of the guild and the broader community of fans. It is essential that the contest of pugilistic craftsmanship take place before an audience, for only the latter can ascertain the worth of the combatants by its very

---

climbin' up a mountain man: when you get to the top you jus' happy, 'kay, so it's like, like you know, when you win a fight, it's like, (very emphatic) it's like *the mission is done*. I trained for this uh, I had a plan to do this an' it worked."

[47]A veteran manager of a dozen boxers makes such principled behavior in everyday life his main criterion of recruitment: "If [a fighter] don't *respect* himself, an' he (adopting a reproachful tone) like to be in bars, he like to be usin' drug, he like to party, well you, *you don't need that fighter*, because you not going nowhere, he can be the bes', but he jus' not going *nowhere*. But you got this kid here, he's not maybe *the greates'*, but (turning laudatory) he *always in the gym*, he's *clean*, he always have his mind clean, you know: he can *go places*, because one day, you gon' to face these two fighters, an' he's a better fighter, but this [one] is in better shape, an' he gon' to win the fight."

[48]Durkheim (1983) lists the "spirit of discipline" as one of the three main components of morality, along with altruism (or group attachment) and autonomy of the will.

presence and collective response. Standing in the public's eye, at the center of attention, having one's name announced, recognized, spoken of, be it in awe or disdain, eliciting the "roar and appreciation of the crowd" is a prized objective and ample gratification in itself. Bernard readily owns up that he boxed "for the *glory*, man: to be seen, the limelight. The limelight. One thin': the limelight. I made it right there in the center of the ring on television, you know. Who can tell you they been on television, like me?"[49] The occupational vernacular acknowledges this in the antinomic contrast it establishes between "marquee fighters" (or "name fighters") and the anonymous "opponents" and "bums" (also called "no-name fighters") who supply so many interchangeable bodies as cannon fodder for better-sponsored peers who are "going somewhere."

Indeed, boxers see themselves as *entertainers* and like to compare their craft to that of performing artists such as movie stars, dancers, and singers for whom the impersonation of character is pivotal and whose stature is set by the compass of their popularity. "I can almost consider myself *an actor almost*," muses Marty, "because I'm tryin' to look good not only for myself but for everyone else an' get the job done, you know what I mean? So yeah, it's almost like an actor, I think that's what actors do, right? They try to impress theirselves an' everyone else." The secret fantasy of my gym buddy Curtis was to become "the Michael Jackson of boxing," that is, to forge a ring personality that would "blossom like a flower throughout the crowd" and enthrall worldwide audiences with stunning exhibitions of grit, tenacity, and fistic virtuosity.

Prizefighting is tailor made for the *personalized construction and public validation of a heroic manly self* because it is a distinctively individualistic form of masculine endeavor whose rules are unequivocal and seemingly place contestants in a transparent situation of radical self-determination. Unlike team sports, where success is of necessity a function of the temperament and actions of others, boxing is a one-on-one clash of virile will and skill in which one depends on nobody and nothing but oneself.[50] Surely, your cornermen assist you during the one-minute intermission between

---

[49]The "limelight" and the public recognition that comes with being active in the ring, in whatever capacity, is also one of the mainsprings behind prolonged careers and comebacks, as Tony indicates: "I'll be hones' with ya, tha's the way, you see all these guys makin' comebacks and stuff like that. It's not the money, it's not the sport, *it's the limelight*. It's the limelight: when you walk inta a place and someone says, (admiringly) 'Hey, there's this person. Hey, that's 'im!' you know, that's what boxin's about I think, as far as a fighter looks at it sometimes."

[50]Fencing and tennis also entail one-on-one competition but confrontation takes place at a distance, through the mediation of specific implements (sword, racquet and ball). Even in wrestling, bodily contact is euphemized by the wearing of uniforms and the contest "feminized" by direct embrace and more rounded, softer gestures. Boxing is virtually unique for the nakedness and frontality of the corporeal clash it commands.

rounds, and their expert advice and support are not without bearing on the fight; but once that bell sounds, you must surrender to the trial of splendid solitary combat. And you cannot turn away, for there is "no place to hide" in the ring. As in the Roman amphitheater where gladiators fought to the death with no possibility of outside succor or recourse, one cannot "feign valor and survive by cowardice" (Barton, 1993) in the squared circle. Correlatively the fighter receives the undivided recognition that befits his fistic deeds, rather than having to share accolades with teammates who may not equally deserve them.

For all these reasons, public vindication of personal fiber and dignity in the ring assumes a strength and purity rarely attained in the outside world, where the struggle for life (and masculine honor) is comparatively ambiguous and uncertain, if not patently biased. What boxers accomplish in the ring, however little it may be, is something that is incontrovertibly theirs and will be theirs for as long as they live—and beyond in the case of the happy few who do become champions, be it at the city, state, or regional level. And whatever their subsequent life course, merely stepping in the ring is a personal acquirement that no authority can snatch from their rightful authorship and ownership.[51]

Boxing offers a theater of controlled peril and virile prowess wherein one can defy the odds and prove oneself publicly in a way that will compel even doubters and detractors to revise their opinion. Many club fighters could make theirs this confidence offered by former heavyweight titlist Leon Spinks (in Berger, 1993, p. 97): "See, my dad said I'd amount to nothing. He would tell people that. And it hurt me to hear him say it. It stayed in my mind. Why'd he say that? What for? Call me a fool out of the blue. Not to my face but to people who'd tell it to me. And that became my thing—to be somebody." The same yearning for recognition is articulated by a 30-year-old journeyman from southern Illinois who walked out on two part-time jobs as pizza delivery man and armoured car driver to apply himself full time to boxing, though his record of 9 defeats in 13 fights hardly presages a rosy future in the business:

---

[51]Looking back over his seven years as a pro after five seasons in the amateurs as he ponders the possibility of retirement, Jeff expresses few regrets about his career, even though he never fulfilled his dream of fighting for a world title: *"It's an accomplishment.* I can look back through my high school years an' say I did this you know, I got these trophies an' awards. I was champion about five different, six different times in the amateurs, open divisions, not novice titles an' uh, I can always go back . . . you're gonna look up [in the local record books] an' it's gonna say *Jeff R-.* An' it never changes, *that's mine, forever.* You can't take it away from me, I've got somethin'. No I didn't play high school football team, an' I wasn't star runnin' back you know, but really who remembers them? I mean that's it, I was the champion, you know: *no one can take that from me—I'll take that to my grave."*

I'm gettin' in the ring 'cause I'm gonna make a believer outa some folks that say I can't do it. That's why. I'm gonna make it, goin' to the top (very quietly, almost meditatively), *startin' at the bottom, goin' to the top, shock Springfield and the world*: everybody be shocked an' everybody be wanna know, how much did you make it, and read it in the paper.

Together, then, the gym and the ring provide a scene in which personal uprightness and merit can be forcefully affirmed and exhibited through skillful and stalwart self-determining action.

Yet it is in the high regard and wide approbation that professional boxers receive from their proximate social milieu that the local morality of pugilism finds its most palpable expression. In their families and neighborhood, fighters are not only revered for their toughness and bravery as noted earlier; they are also hailed for projecting a positive professional image of hard work, discipline, and perseverance. The respect and support they draw is immediately perceptible in the prideful care with which parents treat them and the special attention that friends and associates accord them, in encounters in which acquaintances inquire about an upcoming fight or solicit their commentary on a recently televised bout, and in the gleeful admiration of the children who follow them around or vie to carry their bag on the way to the gym—not to mention those they enlist as new recruits.[52] Pugilists relish being "role models" for other youths and adults around them: What greater affirmation of one's *acceptance in a moral community* could one register than being considered an example for others to emulate?[53] Even drug dealers, this vanguard of the new class of street entrepreneurs in the inner city (Bourgois, 1992; Sánchez-Jankowski, 1993), openly acknowledge the boxer's normative precedence

---

[52]Of all the signs of acclaim he has received, Lorenzo is most proud of making converts: "Through the years of boxin' I done brought up about fifteen guys to d'gym, you know, on an' off, an' everybody respects that an' respects me on d'street where they talk to me about boxin'. An' I give alotta lectures an' I tell 'em how boxin' *help men*, you know how it learned me alot, jus' keeps me off the streets."

[53]"You want kids to look up to you," avers Vinnie, "'cause then you feel that you achieve somethin', you're *somebody*, and bein' a role model, you know you're somebody." Vincent sees it much the same way: "I may not be in the general public's eye, but *there's still somebody out that's watchin' me and looks up to you*, that's whatcha gotta be careful about. And right now I feel I'm a role model, you know. I got *tons* of young nephews and cousins and even, you know, friends and I try to be a role model right now for them. And that's preparing me for one day when I do get into the public's eye and when I've got millions of people lookin' at me." As for Tony, he luxuriates in playing the part of the role model: "Already I think I am, 'cause they all look up to me. These kids ask me for my autograph and everything already. Man, it's really, it's exciting and I always git lil' kids coming up to me all the time."

over them: "They look *up* to me. Because they see, that I jus', I *picked somethin'* an' I *stuck with it* an' I became somethin' an' they look up to me," claims a black light-heavyweight raised in a high-crime area of the city's West Side ghetto on the border of which he is now employed as a hotel night watchman.[54]

Neighbors and kin esteem professional fighters for their stout refusal to bow to social necessity, for fighting—literally—to make a better life for themselves, and for resisting either succumbing to dependency and demoralization as befalls so many ghetto residents or, worse yet, turning to criminal activities as a means of material sustenance and advancement. They are grateful for the fact that, contrary to the sinister figure of the dope seller, the pugilist's industry is oriented, if tenuously, toward the "legit" side of society and adds to the community's commonweal rather than subtracting from it. This is why Rodney enjoys mingling with his "people" during his periodic visits to the South Side from Las Vegas, where he now trains and fights thanks to the financial backing of his manager:

> They look at it as me doin' *somethin' positive*, doin' somethin' *good*, doin' you know, as if I'm tryin' to do, do somethin' *for me, myself*, you know. They see I'm not hangin' out in the streets an' hey, hey! (glowing) they all look up toward me, I'm doin' right, I'm goin' the right route, so. I never take, sell no drugs, or gang-bangin', or none, nonovat in my life.

Matt, who parlayed his pugilistic feats into a steady job as an instructor with the municipal park district, is proud of standing before the teenagers of his "stomping ground" as living proof that one can make it out of the infamous public housing complex of Stateway Gardens through hard work and dutiful abnegation: "I showed them that I lived in the projects, that I was determined, they can be determined too, so they can look forward to that, 'cause you get lots of 'em say 'I wanna be like Matt!'—you can be like Matt, [but] you gotta be dedicated like me."

If for no other reason, boxing is experienced as a positive force in the life of those who make it their career by dint of the *prophylactic function it plays with regard to street crime* and related social ills. Even when they make little or no money and end up in an occupational impasse, shorn of readily transferable skills and useful contacts for

---

[54]One of the great joys of local (i.e., state) champions is to tour the high schools of their neighborhood to exhibit their freshly won title belt and give ritualized speeches on the value of education, the scourge of drugs, and the morality of individual effort.

professional reconversion,[55] the gym and the ring have taken them off the streets and sheltered them for the time being from the dangers there. Thus fighters have at least avoided the worse fates too often visited upon their nonboxing peers and childhood buddies, encapsulated by the macabre triptych of imprisonment, drug abuse or trafficking, and violent death. And they have done so, it appears, through a defiant display of individual volition and moral propriety, as my friend Curtis adduces in this characteristically ornate piece of oration:

> *It's so easy to fuck up, man, and so har' to do good.* I wanna do good, I don't wanna go d'easy way. Boxin' is *d'only way out for me, d'only way.* I know I can go an' steal, sell drugs or kill an' rob people. I don't want that life, Louie, I don't want dat for me. I don't wanna go that route . . . I don't wanna *live dat life, I don't wanna have ta look over my shoulder the rest of my life worryin' 'bout,* somebody talkin' 'bout I sol' 'em dis, I sol' 'em dat n' the police lookin' for me—I just don't want *dat reputation*: I don't wanna be known as (muttered with disdain, with a raucous emphasis on "drug") "Curtis *de drug dealer*" . . . I have seen a lotta ma frien's an' stuff, lotta guys that I be grew up with, tha's been of age before I have, I seen a lotta 'em *use drugs* n' *deal drugs* and did various thin's to try ta fix they habit. Get theyself, you know, some dope, or put some money in they pocket ta try t'take care of theyself. I know tha's the life that they wanted t'live but *I choose* the opposite.

That choosing the profession of prizefighting, and sticking with it in the face of disillusionment and sometimes outright failure, can be a way of asserting their moral superiority over those who opt for—or give in to—the shady trades of the informal economy, is clear upon asking fighters where they would stand today were it not for boxing. The most frequent answer by far points to the malevolent figure of "The Street" and its all-too-familiar procession of joblessness, dereliction, and destruction. "If I wouldn't-a found boxin' I probably would be jus' another one a-them guys on the street," says Dave in a response that condenses the views of many of his compatriots. "I wouldn't-a took nothin' serious at that time uh, it gave me a sense of *responsibility*, a sense of somethin' to do to respect myself an' you know not, not to run the streets an' run in gang

---

[55] The irresolvable dilemma of occupational reconversion from a trade that progressively erodes the very qualifications it requires is beautifully depicted in the moving scene of Ralph Nelson's *Requiem for a Heavyweight* in which retired ring horse "Mountain" Rivera (played by Anthony Quinn) makes a clumsy foray into an employment office only to be compared to a maimed war veteran or a cripple by a well-meaning job placement officer.

fights 'cause it wasn't gettin' me anywhere. . . . I learned that I can go to the gym, fight, learn the trade an' get paid for fightin' than fightin' in the streets an' gettin' nothin'."[56]

Trainers likewise construe their work partly as a civic venture that benefits not only the boxer and his family but the broader society as well. Stoneland's assistant coach Eddie delivers a vibrant sermon on the moral mission of pugilism when queried about what motivates him to clock in daily at the club before going on to take up his shift at the steel mill: "When I come to the gym, *this is my way of fightin' the drugs on d'street an' my way of expressin' myself towar's society deterioratin' teenagers.* . . . 'Cuz I can't go out and just be a vigilante and take a chance on goin' to jail. So this my way of doin' that, you know. And when I come to the gym, I feel that way: I feel I'm *out fightin' all these vices out there.* That's why I put so much in it."[57] As for those who would not need an antidote to the lure of the street, prizefighting offers a (temporary) reprieve and distraction from the drudgery of manual work that would otherwise bring them down to the lowest common denominator of their class—undifferentiated labor power—as Danny makes plain:

If I hadn't found boxin', I be in some trade school as a mechanic or some kind of a laborer, or maybe in a factory. 'Cause that's the only thing for me, (joyfully) I mean, *I'm lucky I found boxin'.* 'Cause you know I'll be (with a touch of bitterness) like the rest of the minorities in Chicago, y'know: jus' workin' in some factory or doin' somethin' laboral to make do.

---

[56]In this regard, boxers are quite representative of their proximate milieu, which remains fundamentally oriented toward the dominant American "focal concerns" of family independence, individual achievement, and material success, notwithstanding recent reports on "race and respectability" in the ghetto based on restaurant chatter and journalistic observation from afar (and without) that have once again refurbished age-old mythologies of "moral collapse" among the (young and bad) black subproletariat, this time under the guise of salvaging the (old and good, if fast declining) traditional black working class.

[57]I could quote pages and pages of interview excerpts on this theme, for the missionary impulse is a leitmotiv of the trainer's occupational culture and self-image. The notion that boxing is a "school of character" that ameliorates society by serving as a crime prevention device has a long pedigree; it is regularly trotted out to counter legal or moral attacks on the manly art. It is not clear that it is founded on more than common sense, since rigorous empirical studies (taking into account selection effects and sampling biases) furnish little evidence that athletic participation in general results in character building, moral development, and good citizenship (Frey & Eitzen, 1991). Nonetheless its ideological function for insiders should not obscure its deeply felt experiential (if not factual) veracity.

No wonder few professional boxers express regrets about entering their bruising trade. Of Chicagoland's 50 pugilists, only 4 hold that they would be better off today had they not embraced the profession of hard knocks, and virtually all reckon that the latter has helped them and enriched their lives.

Coda: A Disquiet and Ambivalent Passion

This paper has sought to draw in rough outline a picture of the pugilistic planet as its main inhabitants see it, or like to imagine it. The resulting sketch is admittedly incomplete and one-sided in that it deliberately accents the beguilements and virtues of prizefighting[58] in an effort to recapture the point of view of the boxer and his grasp—in the double sense of comprehension and embrace—of the fistic occupation as a skilled bodily craft. I have argued that to understand the calling of the pugilist, its allure and resilience, it is not sufficient to identify the (negative) background factors that "push" boxers into the ring from without. One must also, and indeed as a first priority, explicate the (positive) foreground dynamics that "pull" them through the ropes from within and keep them there. For this it is necessary to attend to the lived contours of professional boxing as a self-enclosed moral, emotional, and sensual cosmos in which the skillful and fateful engagement of the trained body offers a "space of forgetting"[59] from restricted everyday lives and a scaffolding for the public erection of a heroic hypermasculine self.

Contrary to Gerald Early's (1991) assertion that boxing is "anti-intelligible," I contend that one can make eminent sense of the seemingly senseless profession of prizefighting, provided one forsakes the view "from the outside looking in" of the detached observer—and the moralizing stance that often derives from scrutinizing a lowly trade from above—to palpate firsthand the tissue and fabric of the boxer's life by submitting oneself in their company to the petty contingencies, calculated risks, and grand illusions to which they are themselves subject. Once we have registered the lure of professional pugilism through the eyes and sentient body of the fighter, the task of analysis becomes one of disassembling the social machinery that

---

[58] A forthcoming companion piece will deal specifically with mechanisms and idioms of exploitation in the pugilistic economy. For a discussion of the realities of risk, injury, and physical debilitation, and how boxers deal with them, see Wacquant (1994a). A thorough summation of the financial, physical, and moral liabilities of prizefighting is Sammons (1988).

[59] This (by way of Nancy Scheper-Hughes) is the apt expression of anthropologist Roberto Da Matta (1983) in his analysis of the place of carnival in Brazilian culture and society.

continually (re)produces this peculiar concatenation of love, rage, and commitment that causes young men from the lower regions of social space to construe and adopt the manly art as a conduit for achieving the dignity and redemption that is otherwise denied them. Put briefly, it consists in explaining the collective genesis and deployment of the *pugilistic libido*, that particular variant of "socially constituted interest" (Bourdieu, 1984) that impels those it inhabits to accord value, and surrender themselves body and soul, to the fistic business.

To recognize that the boxer is linked to his craft by a *quasi-religious relation of giving*[60] is simultaneously to discover how strained and begrudging that devotion is. One does not have to dig very deep to turn up cracks in the wall of pugilistic faith; traces of misgivings and intimations of doubt about it all run like capillaries under the skin of belief. The passion that fastens fighters to their trade does not beget the state of bliss and serenity, the "absolute wealth in feeling" (Hegel's definition of love) they yearn for. Intead, it is shot through with ambivalence and disquietude, even resentment in some quarters. For it is laced with the barely repressed, yet also embodied, knowledge of the dark side of pugilism, what one Chicago pug, in a moment of Freudian candor, calls the "barbarickness" of the sport: the "daily grind" and "torture" that one has to go through in preparation for a fight; the physical abuse that can "make scrambled eggs outa your brains" and the dread of that one punch that will make you "look like Frankenstein for the rest of your life"; the ruthless exploitation that spontaneously brings forth vituperative analogies with slavery and prostitution ("fighters is whores and promoters is pimps, the way I sees it") and threatens to reduce you to a "piece of meat"; the despotic control that small coteries of managers, matchmakers, and promoters—"them with the leather shoes"—exercise over the allocation of the monetary returns of prizefighting.

It is not simply that boxing is "not a well-professionalized occupation," as Ed observes with a studied sense of understatement, in which subterfuge, deception, and treachery are the normal ways of conducting business, a "racket" in which fighters are often treated with the care and consideration befitting "a bar of soap" and where chances of making money are both minuscule and extremely unevenly distributed from the start.[61] Underneath it all, there is the obscure(d) realization that, had one

---

[60]At least at the outset of his career, the commitment that the boxer makes of his body to boxing presents all the characteristics of "the gift" according to Mauss (1950, p. 147): It is "voluntary, so to speak, apparently free and gratuitous, and yet constrained and interested."

[61]However much they strain to believe that the ring is the ultimate locus of meritocracy, fighters cannot ignore that the complex system of patronage and sponsorship that surrounds the ring largely predetermines what happens in it.

not been born near the bottom of society and enjoyed instead the privilege of inheriting an aptitude and liking for school (or even for other less punishing sports), one might have never put on gloves. "Don't nobody be out there fightin' with an MBA, Louie": professional boxers are well aware that their "Cruel Profession" is but a "Poor Boy's Game," to recall the crisp wording of James Baldwin (1963), and thus that theirs is a coerced affection, a *captive love*, one ultimately born of racial and class necessity, though it rises hardly over and against it.[62] "I wish I was born taller, I wish I was born in a rich family, I don't know, wish I was smart, an' I had the brains to go to school an' really become somebody real important," avows Vinnie when asked what he would have liked to change in his life. He is gratified to box "for the people" around him because he hopes it will enable him to give them everything he has lacked so far, and victory in the ring makes him happy beyond compare. Yet he takes sufferance to his own love of boxing: "For me I mean I can't *stand* the sport, I hate the sport, [but] it's carved inside of me so I can't let it go."

No boxer, not even the most successful and entranced of them, is fully immune to the nagging feeling of uneasiness and foreboding rooted in the obdurate fact that those who swipe the monies generated by this extravagant spectacle of disciplined lower-class male fury that is prize-fighting are precisely those who, given the liberty to evolve a truly free love of fighting, did not. In the aftermath of recapturing the heavyweight title in an improbable and epic bout against George Foreman in Kinshasa, Zaire, at the zenith of his success and fame, Muhammad Ali could not forbear this confession (Ali & Durham, 1975, p. 247):

> True, fighting was all I had ever done, but there was always something in me that rebelled against it. Maybe it was because those who profited from it didn't think the fighters as human or intelligent. They saw us as made just for the entertainment of the rich. . . . Then there was this nightmarish image I always had of two slaves in the

---

Thus "protected" boxers (those who, based on a reputation acquired in the amateurs, are granted leeway in selecting inferior opponents to "build up" their record) and run-of-the-mill club fighters (who have to fight whomsoever they get sent against) enter a dual-track system of competition that gives them widely divergent odds of success. And mediocre white pugs, due to the near extinction of their species, look to make considerably more money than more proficient but more populous black and Latino boxers.

[62]Boxers are also evidently called to the ring by the existing structure of gender relations that dictates that ("real") men demonstrate "courage, inner direction, certain forms of aggression, autonomy, mastery," as well as "adventure and considerable amounts of toughness in mind and body" (Patricia Sexton as quoted by Carrigan et al., 1987, p. 75). But, unlike its caste and class counterparts, the gender component of the pugilistic doxa remains unquestioned.

ring. Like in the old slave days on the plantations, with two of us big black slaves fighting, almost on the verge of annihilating each other while the masters are smoking big cigars, screaming and urging us on, looking for the blood.

Finally, the pugilist's love of his craft is tinged with rancor because of the pained awareness, however submerged, that this love will not, indeed *cannot*, be unconditionally reciprocated. For to elevate a chosen few, the Sweet Science of bruising must of necessity deceive and debase the great many, and durably so. And how easy it is to cross the invisible frontier between self-possession and dispossession! Fighters know from experience that boxing "can *hurt* you jus' as bad as it can help you," to quote Vinnie's pithy words again, that "it can make you the best in the world, it can make you the worst in the world." Boxing may uplift you and snatch your existence from the jaws of absurdity and obscurity, but it can just as well push and entrap you further into the very world of marginality and misery from which it beckons to rescue you. Deep within lurks the suspicion, then, that the vista from the top of the mountain of fistic manhood may not be worth the agonizing climb to get there. So the most dedicated and loving boxer cannot but be haunted by the possibility that the enchantment of which he partakes is in truth a curse, and that the bonds of pugilistic love are so many chains that keep him inside a prison of desire and suffering of his very own making: "If I got a regret in boxin'," allows Nate, "I regret puttin' on the first pair of gloves. Now I won't tell you (whining) 'man, I'm sorry I put these gloves on' but if I [had said], (bluntly) 'hey man, I ain't puttin' no gloves on!', that way I wouldn't have that *urge to box*, man: see that urge is hard to get rid of."

In the end, there is no escaping the fact that, whether victorious or vanquished, a boxer leaves bits and pieces of himself in the ring. Every fight, every round, every punch that connects chips away at the living statue of aggrandized virility he is striving to sculpt with the clay of pain, sweat, and blood. At some level, deep down, boxing is horrifying even to fighters (and trainers) and it violates their sense of humanity, though they learn not to feel and show this, including to themselves, as an imperative requirement of their membership in the Durkheimian "church" of prizefighting. The boxer's passion is thus torn asunder by the inescapable contradiction around which the pugilistic planet revolves and which is but one avatar of the contradiction constitutive of all worldly provings of masculinity,[63] namely the demand that fighters erode, nay ruinate, that which it teaches them to value above all else to the point of sacralization: the violent male body, their own and that of their likenesses.

---

[63]"Masculinity is structured through contradiction: the more it asserts itself, the more it calls itself into question" (Segal, 1993, p. 635). Wacquant (1994c) argues this point in the case of bodybuilding.

This is why, for all the affection they vow their craft and the unmatched joys and real benefits it brings them in their own estimation—from dignity, respect, and recognition to discipline, self-confidence, and temporary immunity from the "fast life" of the streets and its hazards—the overwhelming majority of fighters do not wish to see their children march in their footsteps. Over 80% of Chicago's pugilists, roughly the same proportion who see in boxing an escape hatch out of poverty, would prefer that their son not enter the trade. It is also not uncommon for fighters who reach a high level in their profession to try to prevent their younger brother(s) from following their example.[64] And one in four is adamant that he would do everything in his power to abort such an occurrence. Danny enunciates this intuitive, gut-level reticence as well as any of his peers:

No, no, *no fighter wants their son* [to box], I mean you could hear it, you hear it even in Dempsey's age: you never want your son to fight—*that's the reason why you fight, so he won't be able to fight*. . . It's too hard, it's jus' too damn hard. [But you like it, you said you get so much excitement out of it and you don't want to give it up?] Right, but uh, before I got that excitement, I had to pay with a lotta bloody nose, black eyes, uh, there was a lotta pain before I could enjoy that. If he could *hit the books* an' study an' you know, with me havin' a little background in school an' stuff, I could help him. My parents, I never had nobody helpin' me.

If boxers recoil at the idea of exposing their loved ones, the flesh of their own flesh, to the pitiless ordeal of the ring, it is because they know too well, in a sense, everything that they cannot concede because doing so would obliterate the very foundations of their faith in the pugilistic *illusio*. Perhaps only its sacrificial aura and the hope that *others* will recognize and reap the benefits of their participation—"I'm takin' enough punishment for everybody," "I'm doin' it so my son don't gotta do it"— can buttress the belief that this skilled corporeal trade which is *also*, on another level, a gruesome tourney of mutual and self-destruction is worth entering at all.

The boxer's attachment to his craft, then, is a *skewed and malicious passion*, ever tainted by the suspicion that one may be paying too steep a price for the opportunity to make oneself—steeper, at any rate, than anyone who enjoys access to other avenues of ontological realization and social recognition is willing or asked to shoulder. Fighters confusedly comprehend somewhere, somehow, with this sixth sense they have honed risking

---

[64]Thus we have Muhammad Ali and his sibling Ramahan, or Chicago's most successful recent boxer Matt (who won a world title) with his brother Kay (who vegetates as a local journeyman).

their bodies in the ring, that they are, as it were, casualties of their desire for virile brinkmanship. Only by unpacking the logic of boxing's material and moral economy can one hope to disentangle how power and submission, constraint and agency, pleasure and suffering mingle and abet each other in such a manner that prizefighters may be at once their own saviors and their own tormentors.

Dedication

This paper is dedicated to the memory of Vinnie "Nitro" Letizia. He wanted to "become champ of the world and to be financially set so that no one in my family ever has to box or go through hard labor again, and if they want something, my family, my kids, when they get older, they can have it." A motorcycle and a slippery road on a cold winter night decided that he would not be allowed to "go as far as he could to back that dream."

Acknowledgments

This paper is a fragment of a broader study in progress of the culture and economy of pugilism in the ghetto, made possible in part by the financial support of a Lavoisier Fellowship from the French government, the Society of Fellows, and the Milton Fund of Harvard University, and the Russell Sage Foundation.

It benefited from comments and reactions to a related paper on "The Self-Production of Professional Fighters" presented at the New School for Social Research, a lecture on "Boxing as a Durkheimian Social Art" given at the Universidade do São Paulo, and to a talk before the Berkeley Sociology Department. Stimulation also came from the puzzlements and queries of a number of friends and colleagues, among them Janet Abu-Lughod, Michael Kimmel, Nancy Chodorow, Mustapha Emirbayer, Bob Alford, Jeff Manza, and Viviana Zelizer. The ultimate revision took into consideration, however imperfectly, the pointed suggestions of Pierre Bourdieu, Rick Fantasia, and Rogers Brubaker. Robert K. Merton subjected the manuscript to a thorough analytic and stylistic examination that was a learning experience in itself, while Jack Katz raised a wealth (or web) of issues that will require writing a sequel to the present paper.

References

Adler, P.A., & Adler, P. (1991). *Blackboards and backboards: College athletics and role engulfment.* New York: Columbia University Press.

Ali, M., & Durham, R. (1975). *The greatest: My own story.* New York: Random House.

Allen, R. (1991). *Singing in the spirit: African-American sacred quartets in New York City*. Philadelphia: University of Pennsylvania Press.

Appadurai, A. (1988). Putting hierarchy in its place. *Cultural Anthropology*, **3**(1), 36-49.

Ashworth, C.E. (1971). Sport as symbolic dialogue. In E. Dunning (Ed.), *The sociology of sport: A selection of readings*. London: Frank Cass and Co.

Baldwin, J. (1991). The fight: Patterson vs. Liston. In G. Early, *Tuxedo junction: Essays on American culture* (pp. 325-334). New York: Ecco Press. (Original work published in *Nugget*, February 1963).

Barrow, J.L., Jr., & Munder, B. (1988). *Joe Louis: 50 years an American hero*. New York: McGraw-Hill.

Barton, C. (1993). *The sorrow of the ancient Romans: Gladiators and the monster*. Princeton: Princeton University Press.

Berger, P. (1993). *Punch lines*. New York: Four Walls Eight Windows.

Bittner, E. (1973). Techniques and the conduct of social life. *Social Problems*, **30**(3), 249-261.

Bly, R. (1990). *Iron John*. Reading: Addison-Wesley.

Bourdieu, P. (1984). L'intérêt du sociologue. *Economies et société*, 18(October), 12-29.

Bourdieu, P. (1988). Flaubert's point of view. *Critical Inquiry*, **14**, 539-562.

Bourdieu, P. (1993). Comprendre. In P. Bourdieu et al., *La misěre du monde* (pp. 902-938). Paris: Editions du Seuil.

Bourgois, P. (1992). *Homeless in el Barrio: la vie d'un dealer de crack a East Harlem*. Actes de la recherche en sciences sociales, **93**, 59-68.

Brenner, T., with Nagler B. (1981). *Only the ring was square*. Englewood Cliffs, NJ: Prentice-Hall.

Carrigan, T., Connell, B., & Lee, J. (1987). Toward a new sociology of masculinity. *In The making of masculinities: The new men's studies* (pp. 63-100). Boston: Allen and Unwin.

Clément, J.-P. (1987). La force, la souplesse et l'harmonie: étude comparée de trois sports de combat (lutte-judo, aikido). In *Sports et société: Approche socioculturelle des pratiques* (pp.285-301). Paris: Vigot.

Clifford, J. (1991). *The predicament of culture*. Cambridge: Harvard University Press.

Connell, R.W. (1991). Live fast and die young: The construction of masculinity among young working-class men on the margin of the labour market. *Australian and New Zealand Journal of Sociology*, **27**(2), 141-171.

Cooley, C.H. (1966). *Social process*. Carbondale: Southern Illinois University Press. (Original work published 1918).

Csikszentmihalyi, M. (1981). Leisure and socialization. *Perspectives in Biology and Medicine*, **28**(4), 489-497.

Da Matta, R. (1983). An interpretation of Carnival. *Substance*, **37-38**, 162-170.

Davis, G.L. (1985). *I got the word in me and I can sing it, you know: A study of the performed African-American sermon*. Philadelphia: University of Pennsylvania Press.

Durkheim, E. (1983). *L'éducation morale*. Paris: Presses Universitairs de France. (Original work published 1963).

Early, G. (1991). American prizefighter. In *Tuxedo Junction: Essays on American culture* (pp. 171-182). New York: Ecco Press.

Elias, N. (1982). *The civilizing process*. Oxford: Basil Blackwell. (Original work published 1937).

Elias, N., & Dunning, E. (1986). *Quest for excitement: Leisure and sport in the civilizing process*. Oxford: Basil Blackwell.

Emerson, R.M. (1981). Observational field work. *Annual Review of Sociology, 7*, 351-378.

Foley, D.E. (1990). The great American football ritual: Reproducing race, class, and gender identity. *Sociology of Sport Journal, 7*, 11-135.

Freud, S. (1962). *Civilization and its discontents*. New York: W.W. Norton. (Original work published 1930).

Frey, J.H., & Eitzen, D.S. (1991). Sport and society. *Annual Review of Sociology, 17*, 503-522.

Fried, R.K. (1991). *Corner men: Great boxing trainers*. New York: Four Walls Eight Windows.

Fussell, S.W. (1992). *Muscle: Confessions of an unlikely bodybuilder*. New York: Poseidon Press.

Gamson, J. (1994). *Claims to fame: Celebrity in contemporary America*. Berkeley: University of California Press.

Geertz, C. (1979). From the native's point of view: On the nature of anthropological knowledge. In William M. Sullivan & Paul Rabinow (eds.), *Interpretive social science: A reader* (pp. 225-241). Berkeley: University of California Press. (Original work published 1976).

Goffman, E. (1967). Where the action is. In *Interaction ritual* (pp. 149-270). New York: Anchor Books.

Golvin, J.-C. & Landes, C. (1990). *Amphithéatres et gladiateurs*. Paris: Publications du CNRS.

Hauser, T. (1991). *Muhammad Ali: His life and times*. New York: Simon and Schuster.

Heinz, W.C. (1984). *The professional*. Introduction by George Plimpton. New York: Harbor House.

Horowitz, R. (1982). Masked intimacy and urban marginality: Adult delinquent gangs in a Chicago community. *Urban Life, 11*, 3-26.

Katz, J. (1989). *Seductions of crime: Moral and sensual attractions of doing evil*. New York: Basic Books.

Keil, C. (1966). *Urban blues*. Chicago: University of Chicago Press.

Liebling, A.J. (1982). *The sweet science*. London: Penguin Books. (Original work published 1956).

Linhart, R. (1976). *L'établi*. Paris: Editions de Minuit.

Lyng, S. (1990). Edgework: A social psychological analysis of voluntary risk taking. *American Journal of Sociology, 95*(4), 851-886.

Mailer, N. (1971). *King of the hill: On the fight of the century*. New York: New American Library.

Mauss, M. (1950). "Essai sur le don." In *Sociologie et anthropologie* (pp. 143-279). Paris: Presses Universitaires de France. (Original work published 1923).

Merleau-Ponty, M. (1945). *Phénoménologie de la perception*. Paris: Gallimard.

Morrison, R.G. (1986). Medical and public health aspects of boxing. *Journal of the American Medical Association*, **255**, 2475-2480.

Nack, W. (1982, October 18). What's in a name? *Sports Illustrated*, pp. 80-94.

Needleman, C. (1979). *The work of craft*. New York: Knopf.

Pacheco, E. (1992). *Muhammad Ali: A view from the corner*. New York: Birch Lane Press.

Rosaldo, R. (1989). *Ilongot headhunting, 1883-1974: A study in society and history*. Stanford: Stanford University Press.

Rudman, W.J. (1986). The sport mystique in black culture. *Sociology of Sport Journal*, **3**(4), 305-319.

Sammons, J.T. (1988). *Beyond the ring: The role of boxing in American society*. Urbana and Chicago: University of Illinois Press.

Sánchez-Jankowski, M. (1993). *The urban underclass in the United States: Aspects of mobility in the underground economy*. Unpublished manuscript.

Segal, L. (1993). Changing men: Masculinities in context. *Theory and Society*, **22**, 625-642.

Snow, D., & Anderson, L. (1987). Identity work among the homeless: The verbal construction and avowal. *American Journal of Sociology*, **92**, 1336-1371.

Steinross, B., & Kleinman, S. (1989). The highs and lows of emotional labor: Detectives' encounters with criminals and victims. *Journal of Contemporary Ethnography*, **17**, 435-452.

Sullivan, M.L. (1989). *"Getting paid": Youth crime and work in the inner city*. Ithaca: Cornell University Press.

Synnott, A. (1993). *The body social: Symbolism, self, and society*. London and New York: Routledge.

Toperoff, S. (1987). *Sugar Ray Leonard and other noble warriors*. New York: McGraw-Hill.

Veblen, T. (1948). *The portable Veblen*. (David Lerner, Ed.). New York: Viking.

Wacquant, L.J.D. (1992a). The social logic of boxing in black Chicago: Toward a sociology of pugilism. *Sociology of Sports Journal*, **9**(3), 221-254.

Wacquant, L.J.D. (1992b). *Desire, bodily work, and rationality: Practicing and theorizing the craft of boxing*. Lecture presented to the Department of Sociology, University of California at Los Angeles, April 1991.

Wacquant, L.J.D. (1993). *Fatal attraction: The social genesis and meaning of the pugilistic vocation*. Unpublished manuscript, Russell Sage Foundation.

Wacquant, L.J.D. (1994a). A sacred weapon: Bodily capital and bodily labor among professional boxers. In C. Cole, J. Loy, & M.A. Messner

(Eds.), *Exercising power: Making and remaking the body*. Albany: State University of New York Press.

Wacquant, L.J.D. (1994b). The new urban color line: The state and fate of the ghetto in postfordist America. In C.J. Calhoun (Ed.), *Social theory and the politics of identity*. Oxford and New York: Basil Blackwell.

Wacquant, L.J.D. (1994c, in press). Why men desire muscles. *The Body and Society*.

Wacquant, L.J.D. (1994d, in press). Un mariage dans le ghetto. *Actes de la recherche en sciences sociales*.

Wellman, B. (1982). Personal communities. In P.V. Marsden & N. Lin (Eds.), *Social structure and network analysis*. Beverly Hills: Sage.

Wiley, R. (1989). *Serenity: A boxing memoir*. New York: Henry Holt and Company.

Willis, P.; Jones, S.; Canaan, J.; & Hurd, G. (1990). *Common culture: Symbolic work at play in the everyday culture of the young*. Boulder: Westview Press.

PART IV

MAKING PROFESSIONAL BOXING SAFER

This final part of the book is dedicated to examining how professional boxing can be made safer. It looks at professional boxing, compares it with amateur boxing, and makes concrete suggestions for improving the sport.

Chapter 10 turns to a model of medical supervision for professional boxing, the New York State Athletic Commission. Dr. Jordan, the medical director of that commission, recounts the steps that the state of New York has taken to improve safety and prevent major injury to boxers. The program described can be taken as an example for upgrading state supervision of boxing in other states.

The final chapter, written by Dr. Cantu, details and discusses 15 major changes that could dramatically improve safety in professional boxing. Eight of the suggestions come from the AMA's advisory panel; the rest are ones Dr. Cantu has developed while working with others to improve the safety of boxing. These suggestions form a working document for those who wish to work to improve the lot of professional boxers.

Professional Boxing: Experience of the New York State Athletic Commission

Barry D. Jordan

Unlike amateur boxing, professional boxing lacks a national regulatory agency that will ensure the uniformity of rules and regulations throughout the United States. Accordingly, professional boxing is regulated on the local or regional level by state boxing or athletic commissions. The New York State Athletic Commission (NYSAC) has been in the forefront of medical safety in boxing and is the prototype of a state boxing commission. This chapter outlines the medical experiences of the NYSAC in relation to medical safety in boxing.

Functions of the New York State Athletic Commission

The NYSAC governs all professional boxing in the state of New York. Its primary function is to determine whether or not a boxer is physically fit to participate in boxing. The NYSAC is also responsible for providing medical coverage at all boxing matches conducted in the state. Each ringside physician approved by the NYSAC must attend a detailed training course on the medical aspects of boxing, which includes the recognition and management of acute and chronic neurologic injury.

In addition to the ringside physician, the NYSAC also has the Medical Advisory Board (MAB), which consists of physicians of various medical specialties. The panel's functions are to provide recommendations to maximize safety in boxing and to approve medical doctors to work as ringside physicians. Furthermore, the MAB may assist in determining the necessity and duration of medical suspension for boxers that exhibit unusual medical circumstances.

Medical Preparticipation Screening

Before an individual is licensed to box professionally in New York State, he must have a detailed physical and neurological examination, an electrocardiogram (EKG), a computed tomography (CT) scan, an electroencephalogram (EEG), and a dilated eye examination by an ophthalmologist. These tests are repeated on an annual basis. Table 10.1 shows the number of boxers licensed in New York State from 1988 through 1991. An average of 325 boxers were licensed annually from 1988 through 1990. The drop in 1991 occurred because of a temporary decrease in the number of shows.

Table 10.2 shows the number of abnormal medical screening tests among licensed professional boxers in New York State during 1988 through 1991. It includes the CT scan, EEG, EKG, and eye examination.

During the four-year period, 11 boxers were denied licenses on the basis of an abnormal CT scan (Table 10.3). On an annual basis the frequency of

Table 10.1 Boxers Licensed in New York State from 1988 to 1991

1988	1989	1990	1991
335	332	309	169

Table 10.2 Abnormal Medical Screening Tests Among Licensed Boxers in New York State (1988-1991)

Test	1988		1989		1990		1991	
	No.	%	No.	%	No.	%	No.	%
CT	3	.9	3	.9	2	.6	3	1.8
EEG	10	3.0	15	4.5	7	2.3	4	2.4
EKG	12	3.6	2	.6	2	.6	8	4.7
Eye exam	19	5.7	11	3.3	3	1.0	4	2.4

Table 10.3 Types of Abnormalities Found in Computed Tomography (CT) Scans

Type of abnormality	No. of boxers
Focal hypodense lesions	8
Basal ganglia	4
Frontal lobe	2
Occipital lobe/thalamus	1
Cerebellum	1
Arachnoid cysts	2
Middle fossa	1
Suprasellar cistern	1
Focal hyperdense lesion	1
Frontal lobe	1

boxers with abnormal CT scans was less than 2%. This frequency of abnormal CT scans is lower than that previously reported (1) because atrophy alone would not preclude a boxer from obtaining a license if his neurological examination was normal. The most common abnormality on CT scan was focal hypodense lesions that were felt to be suggestive of posttraumatic encephalomalacia or infarction. The basal ganglia were the most frequent area in which focal hypodense lesions were seen to occur. Two boxers with arachnoid cysts were denied licenses because of the potential risk of hemorrhage into these cysts. One boxer exhibited a focal hyperdense lesion that was consistent with intracerebral calcification or hemorrhage.

Over the four-year period, 36 boxers had abnormal EEGs. On an annual basis this averages less than 5% per year. The most common EEG abnormality was focal in nature (20 cases), followed by diffuse (8 cases) and paroxysmal (8 cases) features. The majority of focal abnormalities were characterized as either frontal/temporal or multifocal slowing. Boxers with diffuse abnormalities tended to exhibit diffuse slowing or poor background organization, or both.

Over the four-year period, 24 boxers had abnormal EKGs. The most frequent abnormality was ST segment/T wave changes consistent with ischemia (10 cases). Six boxers had EKGs that were suggestive of a previous myocardial infarction. Premature ventricular contractions were noted in four boxers, and three boxers exhibited third-degree atrial-ventricular block. One boxer had atrial premature contractions. Overall, the annual incidence of abnormal EKGs among boxers remained less than 5%.

An annual dilated eye examination by an ophthalmologist is required for all boxers in New York State. During the years 1988 through 1991, a total of 37 boxers had abnormal eye examinations. The ocular pathologies noted among these 37 boxers are shown in Table 10.4. The annual incidence of boxers having an abnormal eye examination ranged between 1% and 6%. Retinal tears and retinal holes were the most commonly noted ocular pathology (12 cases each). Cataracts were the third most common pathology noted. Only four retinal detachments and two vitreous detachments were observed over the four-year period.

General Bout Statistics

In 1988, 189 professional bouts were conducted in New York State (Table 10.5). Four-round bouts were the most frequently scheduled type of competition, followed by 10-round bouts. Six- and eight-round bouts each accounted for 15% of all the scheduled bouts. Only four bouts were for 12-15 rounds.

Among the 189 bouts, 122 resulted in a T.K.O. or K.O. (Table 10.6). The frequency of T.K.O./K.O. was lowest for 4-round bouts (Table 10.7), and all of the 12- to 15-round bouts resulted in a T.K.O. or K.O. (Table 10.7).

Table 10.4 Types of Abnormal Eye Findings

Type of abnormality	No. of boxers
Retinal tears	12
Retinal holes	12
Cataracts	5
Retinal detachments	4
Vitreous detachments	2
Increased intraocular pressure	1
Radial keratotomy	1
Hypoplasia of optic nerve	1
Decreased visual acuity	1

Table 10.5 Distribution of Professional Bouts in New York State (1988) by Number of Rounds

4 rounds		6 rounds		8 rounds		10 rounds		12-15 rounds	
No.	%	No.	%	No.	%	No.	%	No.	%
71	38	29	15	28	15	57	30	4	2

Table 10.6 Distribution of Outcomes of Professional Bouts in New York State (1988)

Knock-out		Technical knock-out		Decisions		Draws		Disqualification	
No.	%	No.	%	No.	%	No.	%	No.	%
19	10	103	54	59	31	7	4	1	1

Table 10.7 Number of Bouts Resulting in T.K.O./K.O. in New York State (1988) by Rounds

4 rounds		6 rounds		8 rounds		10 rounds		12-15 rounds	
No.	%	No.	%	No.	%	No.	%	No.	%
36	51	21	72	21	75	40	70	4	100

Bouts scheduled for 6-10 rounds had a T.K.O./K.O. frequency of 70%-75%. Of all T.K.O./K.O.s, 80% occurred within the first three rounds. T.K.O./K.O.s were most frequent in the first round (Figure 10.1). Only one T.K.O./K.O. occurred after the ninth round.

Medical Injuries

Ringside physicians in New York State are required to complete injury report forms on any boxer sustaining an injury in the ring. This includes any boxer that loses a bout on the basis of a T.K.O. or K.O. Unless otherwise specified, boxers who experience a loss secondary to a T.K.O. or K.O. are classified as having a craniocerebral injury.

During the four-year period under observation there were a total of 574 medical injuries (Table 10.8). The most common injury was craniocerebral; the overwhelming majority of these craniocerebral injuries was minor concussions that were not associated with loss of consciousness or prolonged postconcussive symptoms. Among the 218 non-craniocerebral injuries, facial lacerations were by far the most common (133 cases). These were followed by hand injuries (29 cases). Acute eye injuries (7 cases) were relatively uncommon in New York State. This is partially attributable

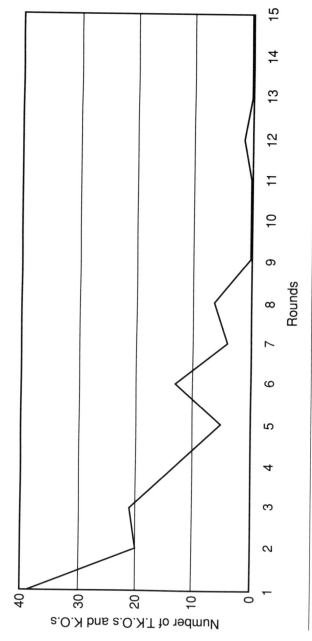

Figure 10.1 Distribution of 122 technical knockouts (T.K.O.s) and knockouts (K.O.s) by round of occurrence.

Table 10.8 Types of Medical Injuries Among Professional Boxers in New York State (1988-1991)

Type of injury	No. of boxers
Craniocerebral	**356**
Non-craniocerebral	**218**
Facial laceration	133
Hand	29
Eye	7
Exhaustion	7
Abdomen	7
Nose	7
Shoulder	5
Ear	5
Rib/thorax	5
Elbow	4
Forearm	2
Mandible	2
Ankle	2
Muscle	1
Hematuria	1
Knee	1

Table 10.9 Injury Rates[a] of Common Injuries Among Professional Boxers in New York State (1988-1991)

Type of injury	1988	1989	1990	1991
Craniocerebral	33.4	34.9	59.0	21.9
Non-craniocerebral	17.6	19.0	20.7	18.9
Facial laceration	8.7	13.6	12.9	11.2
Hand injury	1.2	0.6	4.9	4.7

[a]Injury rates per 100 boxers.

to the utilization of the thumbless or thumb-locked boxing glove that is designed to prevent thumbing injuries to the eye.

Table 10.9 demonstrates the injury rates for the more common medical injuries encountered by professional boxers in New York State. For craniocerebral injuries the rate ranged between 21.9 and 59 per 100 boxers. This resulted in an average annual incidence of 37.3 craniocerebral injuries per 100 boxers. Despite this frquency of craniocerebral injuries, only one death occurred during the four-year period. For the non-craniocerebral injuries the average annual incidence was 19.1 per 100 boxers. The annual incidence rate of facial lacerations ranged between 8.7 and 13.6 per 100 boxers. Of interest is the fact that there was a fourfold increase in the incidence of hand injuries between 1988 and 1991. The etiology of this phenomenon is uncertain, but could conceivably reflect changes in the methods of hand wrapping or the manufacturing of boxing gloves, or both.

Medical Suspensions

There are several indications for the medical suspension of a boxer in New York State. One indication is the boxer's having sustained a medical injury. In New York, boxers who sustain a T.K.O. or K.O. secondary to cerebral concussion are suspended, anywhere from 45 to 60 days for a T.K.O. and 90 days for a K.O. (2). These boxers must have a repeat CT scan and EEG before they can be medically reinstated. For all other noncerebral injuries, boxers are usually suspended until their injuries have healed. During the period of observation, seven boxers were suspended indefinitely pending a neurological or medical evaluation after a boxing competition. The majority of the cases were boxers who experienced a concussion associated with profound or prolonged postconcussive symptoms.

A second indication for medical suspension in New York State is poor performance. It is the policy and opinion of the NYSAC medical department that poor performance predisposes a boxer to injury. Accordingly, boxers who experience six consecutive losses or three consecutive losses by T.K.O. or K.O. are medically suspended (2). During the years 1988 through 1991, eight boxers were suspended for consecutive losses. Another boxer was medically suspended because he demonstrated inferior boxing skills that might predispose him to significant medical injury.

Another indication for medical suspension in New York State is evidence of progressive neurological deterioration. Two boxers demonstrated progressive ataxia and slurring of speech consistent with chronic neurologic injury (CNI) associated with boxing (3, 4). Another boxer was suspended on the basis of progressive atrophy and posttraumatic encephalomalacia associated with boxing (5).

Conclusion

The NYSAC is the prototype of a state boxing commission and is in the forefront for medical safety in boxing. The NYSAC's primary concern is the health and protection of the boxer. Medical supervision and regulation in New York State are maximized by the utilization of properly trained ringside physicians and the MAB. Medical preparticipation screening plays an instrumental role in assuring that boxers who enter the ring are medically fit and physically capable of competitive professional boxing. Severe medical injuries are rare in New York State, and boxers that exhibit untoward effects of boxing are medically suspended. Further clinical research is indicated to promote medical safety in boxing.

References

1. Jordan, B.D.; Jahre, C.; Hauser, W.A.; Zimmerman, R.D.; Zarelli, M.; Lipsitz, E.C.; Johnson, V.; Warren, R.F.; Tsairis, P.; Folk, F.S. Computed tomography in 338 professional boxers. Radiology 185:509-512; 1992.
2. New York State Athletic Commission. Laws and rules regulating boxing and wrestling matches 1992-1993. New York: New York Sate Athletic Commission; 1993.
3. Jordan, B.D. Neurologic injury in boxing. Hosp. Med. 27(4):93-105; 1991.
4. Jordan, B.D. Chronic Neurologic Injuries in Boxing. In: Jordan, B.D., ed. Medical aspects of boxing. Boca Raton, FL: CRC Press; 1993, pp. 177-185.
5. Jordan, B.D.; Jahre, C.; Hauser, W.A.; Zimmerman, R.D.; Peterson, M. Serial computed tomography among professional boxers. J. Neuroimaging 2:181-185; 1992.

CHAPTER 11

How to Make
Professional Boxing Safer

Robert C. Cantu

Through the 1962 "Statement on Boxing" of the AMA Committee on the Medical Aspects of Sports, the AMA long ago addressed the issue of the medical risks of boxing (1). It was the January 14, 1983, issue of the *Journal of the American Medical Association (JAMA)* that sparked a debate resulting in extensive major network television coverage, newspaper articles and editorials, magazine stories, an AMA-sponsored conference on the medical aspects of boxing, a Congressional hearing on boxing, and the embarrassing position of the AMA appearing to support both sides of the debate simultaneously.

In the January 14, 1983, issue of *JAMA* were two major articles on boxing (2, 3), neither calling for its abolition, and two impassioned editorials calling for the abolition of boxing on moral, ethical, and medical grounds (4, 5). It is ironic that the AMA's Council on Scientific Affairs study on the safety issues of boxing, a study and recommendations already approved by the House of Delegates at the 1982 annual meeting and thus the official policy of the AMA, appears in the same issue as the conflicting editorial opinions. The council, after deliberation on the medical evidence, concluded that "boxing is a dangerous sport and can result in death or long-term brain injury" but that to ban boxing would not be a "realistic solution to the problem of brain injury" (3; p. 256). It called for establishing a national registry for all amateur and professional boxers, mandating the use of uniform protective equipment and standardizing ringside safety and medical procedures.

At odds with these recommendations was the editorial of Lundberg, who concluded, "Boxing seems to me to be less sport than is cockfighting; boxing is an obscenity. Uncivilized man may have been bloodthirsty. Boxing, as a throwback to uncivilized man, should not be sanctioned by any civilized country" (4; p. 250). Furthermore, a second editorial by Van Allen chimed in, "Is now not the time to suppress exposure of this fragment of our savagery by the mass media and leave boxing to those who enjoy privately staged dogfights?" (5; p. 251).

While the controversy raged, the AMA conference on the medical aspects of boxing was held in February of 1983. The panel, which included professors of neurology and neurosurgery, reviewed all the medical evidence and did not call for a ban on boxing; instead, it made eight recommendations to improve boxing safety.

At the June 1983 AMA annual meeting in Chicago the 351-member House of Delegates adopted by voice vote a resolution calling for the "elimination of boxing from amateur scholastic, intercollegiate, and government athletic programs" because it is deleterious to health. This June resolution represents the first time the AMA officially opposed boxing and conflicts with previous endorsement expressed in the Council on Scientific Affairs report. The AMA, apparently not for the first time, was endorsing conflicting policies. When asked about this dilemma, AMA spokesperson Mike Cherskov responded that "he didn't know whether the June resolution accurately represented the feelings of most physicians . . . and that the board of trustees traditionally endorses reports of its scientific committee."

Let us now review 15 proposed points for the improvement of safety in boxing, especially professional boxing. They include the recommendations of the AMA's Council on Scientific Affairs as well as others that appear cogent to this author.

1. Establish a national registry of all professional boxers. In amateur boxing there is a national passport registry system in which each boxer has a "passport" containing all the pertinent medical and boxing exposure information on the athlete. A similar national registry is sorely needed in professional boxing. The medical restrictions concerning eligibility to box must also become uniform nationally. This would eliminate the present practice of a fighter medically barred in one state fighting in another state under an assumed name.

This author feels we also need not only a national boxing registry or commission, but a strong-willed, honest national boxing commissioner comparable to commissioners in other major sports.

Others in professional boxing agree. To quote nationally renowned trainer Teddy Atlas:

We need a national commission or some way of having consistent blanket control and knowledge of all fighters, so as to avoid fighters

K.O.d one night in a city fighting two nights later in another. It's not the [state] commissioners' fault they don't have the money or have the means to handle the situation without federal money. What of course scares me is that a national federally subsidized commission means political cronies that know nothing and don't care, but maybe that's the nature of the beast when you venture into national commissions.

The first attempt to introduce a federal boxing bill was made in 1961 by then Senator Estes Kefauver. Through the years other attempts have been made, but the 1993 bills introduced by Senator William Roth (S1189) and Representative William Richardson (HR2607) are gaining momentum. For the first time a boxing bill in the House and Senate have the same content and bipartisan backing. The salient features of the Professional Boxing Corporation Act of 1993 include the following:

Objective: Establish a Professional Boxing Corporation to help

1. create a universal set of rules and regulations governing boxing;
2. eliminate exploitation, conflicts of interest, questionable judging, corruption, and the influence of organized crime; and
3. safeguard the health and welfare of boxers and establish the sport's credibility.

Administration: An executive director will be appointed by the President of the United States. The director will name a professional boxing board of 5 members who will establish a Congress of State Boxing Administrators.

Some of the Corporate Functions:

1. Establish a national registry and licensing data base.
2. Issue certificates of licensing and registration.
3. Prescribe regulations to ensure safety of participants.
4. Establish standards.
5. Encourage insurance funds for the boxing community.
6. Prescribe regulations prohibiting conflicts of interest.

Steve Acunto, who with Rocky Marciano cofounded The American Association for the Improvement of Boxing (AAIB), has this to say:

The PBC Bill sponsored by this committee has the best potential to date to solve the problem of sound regulation, especially since it will be self-supporting and portends no cost to the taxpayer.

It is ludicrous and reprehensible to think that our great country has not been able to regulate boxing and restore public confidence through an organization that would place it on the same plane as other major sports in America. This undertaking will not succeed unless individuals appointed to PBC are truly knowledgeable, competent, and dedicated to achieving the purposes of the bill. The primary purpose should be the physical safety and financial security of the pugilists who are now victims of poor regulations.

All of us here should be inspired by the magnificent mosaic of the Olympic athletes who exemplify the true integrity of the sport. We cannot let them down by permitting unscrupulous individuals to prevail on the American boxing scene.

Boxing is at the crossroads. Today, the world's oldest sport is fighting to survive a seemingly endless chain of corruption, fragmentation, and disarray which has left it at a hopeless impasse. That's why new legislation proposed by Senators William Roth and William Richardson and backed by Senator John Glenn is of vital importance and deserves the support of everyone concerned with the survival of the game. The Roth Bill would create a non-profit Professional Boxing Corporation, while Richardson's legislation would establish a U.S. Boxing Commission under the U.S. Department of Labor. The resulting Professional Boxing Corporation (PBC) will be completely self-supporting except for an initial start-up load which will be paid back with interest—at absolutely no cost to the taxpayer. Further, the PBC will not supplement any state boxing regulations nor will it attempt to micro-manage professional boxing. Boxing will be—as it should be—left to boxing.

The proposed Professional Boxing Act of 1993 has been carefully screened by the AAIB, and we would like to state unequivocally that the Roth-Richardson bills are the best yet devised as a permanent solution to upgrading boxing and placing it on the level of other major professional sports.

For skeptics who say, "I've heard that song before," we understand your cynicism. Since the first boxing bill was introduced in 1961, there have been no less than eight bills or hearings designed for the same purpose with an almost identical litany. *Hearings, testimonies of champions, promoters and ring participants* . . . followed by a universal clarion call for *"Cleaning up boxing"* and *establishing a national governing body.* But, in the end, the result has always been, to paraphrase the Great Bard, "full of sound and fury, and signifying nothing . . . zilch . . . nada!"

Despite this past history, this new legislation may indeed be *the* breakthrough, but it won't be a reality without the support of everyone concerned with the survival of boxing. We urge everyone connected with the sport, including boxers, managers, trainers, sports writers, and publishers of ring publications, to join us in expressing support for Bill #S2852, which will establish the Professional Boxing Corporation.

There never was a better time to say "enough" to boxing's corruption, inadequate protection for the ring combatants, and lack of confidence in the fight game. Public support, coupled with the boxing writers of America, will make this bill a reality.

2. Authorize the ringside physician to stop or terminate bouts. In most states it presently is up to the discretion of the referee to suspend action to seek the ringside physician's opinion as well as to terminate a contest. In my opinion, the ringside physician should also have those powers, and if there is disagreement, the physician should be empowered to override the referee. Who should know better when to suspend or terminate action—a properly trained, experienced ringside physician, or a well-intentioned but not necessarily medically trained referee?

3. Hold frequent medical training seminars for ring personnel. In many states, becoming a ringside physician only requires a license to practice medicine. It does not require that you be a neurologist or neurosurgeon or have had extensive experience dealing with head injuries. This is wrong, as all ringside physicians should be experienced in the recognition and initial assessment of head and other injuries. All ringside personnel should be instructed in Basic Life Support (BCLS), and the physician ideally in Advanced Life Support (ACLS).

4. Provide adequate ringside life support systems and evacuation plans. State-of-the-art emergency (EMT) personnel and equipment should be at ringside. Plans should be made for evacuation to a neurosurgical facility where a neurosurgeon is on duty and available.

5. Boxing matches should be held only when proper neurosurgical facilities are nearby. Matches should not be held in remote locations where full neuroradiologic and neurosurgical capabilities are not immediately available. To do otherwise is to needlessly risk fatal injury before diagnostic medical care can be rendered. Some have advocated the ringside attendance of a neurosurgeon. To me this is like a priest at a hanging; it may provide comfort, but it will not alter the outcome. A neurosurgeon is only of value where he or she works, in the hospital, and no match should occur without immediate access to neurosurgical care. This is especially true when we consider the second impact syndrome or an acute subdural hematoma, which can place the athlete in a life-threatening situation within minutes.

6. Establish mandatory safety standards for ringside equipment. A boxer may receive a brain injury not only from an opponent's direct blow, but also indirectly from having his head strike a ring post or the floor. Uniform safety standards regarding all ring equipment, the padded floor surface, the tension and number of ring ropes, and the padding on ring posts should be established and adopted.

7. Upgrade and enforce the medical evaluation of boxers by state boxing commissions. Just as amateur boxers in this country do, professionals should undergo standardized periods of enforced inactivity after bouts terminated by head blows. As is true in New York State, there should be periodic examinations and criteria for when a head CT or MRI scan should be done.

Each professional boxer also should have his own psychological profile established with a battery of psychological tests. It is imperative to have such standardized testing on a national basis. If deterioration consistent with brain injury is determined, a boxer should be withheld from the ring, both sparring and contests. Neither boxing fans nor boxers themselves wish professional boxers to sustain permanent and progressive brain injury, and it is apparent today that such injury can usually be detected by neuropsychological tests before atrophy or other chronic traumatic brain injury is seen on head CT or MRI scans.

8. Eliminate all "Tough Man" contests. Tough Man contests, no-holds barred boxing with no weight classes, are already illegal in many states. This activity should be banned everywhere. This is the opinion of both the AMA's panel of experts and myself. This activity is not boxing and does not sufficiently protect the safety of the combatants. To this author, it is analogous to the state of affairs the AMA editors have falsely ascribed to professional boxing.

Although embellished by my personal opinions, the previously outlined eight proposals were all recommended by the AMA's panel of experts. Now let us turn to some additional suggestions I believe would further enhance the safety of boxing, especially at the professional level, where it is most sorely needed.

9. Use better criteria to select ringside physicians. In most states the selection of ringside physicians is largely a political process, more a question of who you know rather than what you know. Often ringside physicians have no special training in the immediate assessment and care of head injuries, the most life-threatening condition they are likely to face. This is just plain wrong.

Boxing physicians should be selected from the elite of sports medicine physicians. All must have specialized training and experience in the recognition of head injuries, especially mild concussions. They must fully understand when it is prudent to stop a contest because of head blows.

10. Do not allow the round-ending bell to save a boxer from a knockout. If a boxer is rendered unconscious or is still stunned (Grade 1 concussion) and unable to continue with less than 10 seconds left in a round, the referee's knockout or "standing" count should continue. If it reaches 10, the fight should be over. Boxers should not be able to be "saved by the bell."

This is especially important when we reflect on the fact that the Second Impact Syndrome not only is more common than previously thought, but also occurs not just in football, but in all contact and collision sports, including boxing. Thus all ringside physicians must be acutely aware of this condition. (See chapter 3 for a description of the Second Impact Syndrome.) With such a catastrophic condition, for which the mortality rate may approach 50% and the chance of morbidity is nearly 100%, prevention takes on the utmost importance. Prevention is clearly the key. To allow a boxer who has already sustained a concussion to continue because the "bell saved him" is to invite this condition.

11. Suspend for a specified period boxers rendered unconscious or in bouts terminated due to head blows. This is especially important because of concerns related to the Second Impact Syndrome. Suspensions such as those for amateur boxing would be prudent:

- 30 days' suspension: The contest is stopped due to minor head blows or excessive standing eight counts.
- 90 days' suspension: The boxer is unresponsive for less than two minutes, or the boxer has been given multiple 30-day suspensions in the same year.
- 180 days' suspension: The boxer is unresponsive for more than two minutes.

Before resuming boxing after a restriction, the boxer must be free of all postconcussion symptoms and have a physician's examination and clearance to return. Furthermore, a boxer may be required to have an EEG or CT scan at the examining physician's discretion.

As discussed in chapter 10, presently in New York State a professional boxer stopped by a T.K.O. is suspended for 45 to 60 days and by a K.O. for 90 days. All such boxers must have a CT scan or EEG before they can be reinstated.

12. Apply the same suspensions and medical clearance restrictions for sparring as for competition. The brain does not respond differently to injuries sustained in the gym versus a formal contest. Thus the rules regarding suspension after head injury should be the same.

It is interesting to reflect on the words of renowned trainer Teddy Atlas (personal communication):

It has been my experience and the feeling of my teacher Cus D'Amato, who spent 50 years in the sport, that many times when there is a serious injury such as hemorrhaging of the brain automatically it is assumed that the condition was the result of those punches from the immediate fight. Cus' feeling was that in his investigations of these incidents he found that many of the fights were boring, uneventful fights where few punches were landed yet [they ended with] the tragic result. His findings were that the fighters had suffered a previous undisclosed injury that went unreported or possibly a cerebral aneurysm was present. But without the benefit of an autopsy in the tragic cases where death occurred, the conclusion that punches in the fight caused the condition was unfair and inaccurate.

Ted goes on to say regarding the risk of injury to a boxer: "If there is injury risk it is obviously to a great extent during his sparring in the gym, since he's doing much more sparring than rounds of fighting. So there should be some commission supervision (if you can find qualified people). If a guy is hurt or K.O.d in the gym it should be known."

13. <u>Improve coaching and possibly certify trainers and managers.</u> At the top of the list of ways to improve safety in the sport for Teddy Atlas is "better coaching so the fighters are taught what the real approach of the sport is supposed to be—*hit and don't get hit* as much as possible. I don't know how practical it really can be but *screen* and *rate* and *test* the coaches and get rid of the unqualified—they're dangerous."

I believe these are very cogent words whose time has come. It doesn't require great prescience to realize that improper coaching of a boxer invites injury.

14. <u>Improve and certify boxing equipment.</u> Everything that was included in the sixth recommendation regarding ring equipment also applies to the boxer's equipment. It is ridiculous to think that the bicycle, hockey, motorcycle, and football gear worn by children must pass rigid certification standards before it can be sold, yet there are no certification standards or process for boxing headgear. An offshore country can produce boxing headgear under no standards or controls, import it to this country where an American label may be stuck on, and sell it. This is wrong. The same comprehensive research that was conducted to certify football helmets, for example, should be carried out for protective boxing headgear.

Boxing gloves, like headgear, are archaic and much in need of space-age materials and technology. Presently their weight can be significantly increased by sweat and water absorbed by the leather. The padding can also remold during the course of a fight and provide less of an impact cushion over the knuckles as the fight progresses.

15. <u>Continue research on chronic brain injury.</u> This final recommendation for boxing also pertains to other contact/collision sports. The research started by the Johns Hopkins study on amateur boxing as described in chapter 4 should be continued and extended to other sports in which head contact is common. Recent articles have appeared regarding chronic brain injury in soccer, football, rugby, and the equestrian sports, to name a few. Other sports in which the overall risk of head injury is low have unique positions or events (such as the goalie in soccer or the pole vaulter in track) where the risk of head injury may be high. All studies in other sports presently lack controls, which also was true of all the boxing studies prior to the Johns Hopkins study.

We need more sophisticated neuropsychiatric tests that one would hope could be administered within 15 minutes. We also must develop more accurate brain scanning devices that will detect not only early structural but also physiological changes.

Therefore, to make not only boxing but all sports with a risk of head injury safer, significant research challenges lie ahead for the sports medicine/sport science community.

References

1. American Medical Association Committee on the Medical Aspects of Sports. Statement on boxing. JAMA 181:242; 1962.
2. Ross, R.J.; Cole, M.; Thompson, J.S.; Kim, K.H. Boxers—computed tomography, EEG and neurological evaluation. JAMA 249:211-213; 1983.
3. Council on Scientific Affairs. Brain injury in boxing. JAMA 249:242-257; 1983.
4. Lundberg, G.D. Boxing should be banned in civilized countries. JAMA 249:250; 1983.
5. Van Allen, M.W. The deadly degrading sport. JAMA 249:250-251; 1983.

CONCLUSION

So the question remains: Should boxing be banned or supported?

Boxing is inarguably a risky sport. Part II clearly shows that it entails the possibility of brain damage, eye injury, and harm to other parts of the body. But it remains true that the risks inherent in boxing are also found in a number of other contact and collision sports that society condones, such as football, soccer, horse racing, and many other adventurous sports like skydiving and hang gliding.

Boxing also has sociological significance. The sport affords the small, short, lightweight athlete from a low socioeconomic background the opportunity to "be somebody." Golf, tennis, and fencing aren't options for inner city youths. In fact, studies have shown that amateur boxers are better educated and work in higher occupations than their parents or siblings (1). And, as is clearly pointed out by Dr. Wacquant in chapter 9, boxing can provide a meaningful direction to the lives of ghetto residents, as well as providing them some respect from their communities (which also ensures some personal safety).

There also is the question whether it is morally justified to take away the right of people to box without overwhelmingly conclusive justification. If we agree with the argument of Dr. Wildes in chapter 8, a society such as ours, with no common ground for making moral decisions, limits the government's justification for restricting the liberty of its citizens to engage in the sport.

One area worth focusing on in this debate is the difference between amateur and professional boxing. As Dr. Estwanik demonstrates in chapter 2, many safety precautions have been taken in amateur boxing that are absent in professional boxing. The results of the study done by Drs. Stewart and Gordon described in chapter 4 may be in part attributable to these safety restrictions. However, professional boxing, in my opinion, is not sport but rather big-business entertainment. In professional boxing it's not just winning, but how the athlete wins and the size of the crowds he can draw that determine his career. This often has meant a lack of concern for the safety and well-being of the professional boxer.

To me, though, this doesn't mean we should throw out professional boxing. Boxers have the right to participate in professional boxing, knowing the risks, in order to possibly achieve an economic security they might never otherwise reach. This is especially true when society condones sports such as motorcycle, car, and horse racing, pursuits with more than a tenfold greater chance of fatality than boxing, and football, which leads to more than 250,000 concussions annually and more than 95% of all catastrophic sports injuries (2). What I do support is the safety measures enumerated in chapters 10 and 11 to improve the sport.

Boxing, and in particular professional boxing, must be made safer for participants. It should follow the lead of football, in which the rising incidence of quadriplegia and serious head injury spurred a variety of corrective changes in 1976. These changes resulted in an 80% reduction in subdural hematoma, the major cause of death, and nearly a sixfold reduction in quadriplegia, the major type of catastrophic disability (3). Now is not the time to ban boxing, but rather to take corrective action that will enhance safety and protect the interests of the participants. Physicians, whether they assist directly at ringside as described in chapter 7 or just support legislation and reforms in boxing, can play a large role in accomplishing this.

References

1. Blondstein, J.L.; Clark, E. Further observations on the medical aspects of amateur boxing. Br. Med. J. 1:362; 1957.
2. Cantu, R.C. Catastrophic injuries in high school and collegiate athletes: a five year experience 1982-1987. Surgical Rounds for Orthopaedics 11:62-66; 1988.
3. Cantu, R.C.; Mueller, F.O. Catastrophic football injuries in the USA (1977-1990). Clin. J. Sport Med. 2:180-185; 1992.

Index